Dedication

This book was written because of my wife Sue, and for her. Without her none of it would have been possible. Nor would any of my life have made sense.

To all those wonderful people whom we met, and for the help which they gave to us in so many different ways, thank you.

I hope that we gave back as much as we received.

M.H.H.

My thanks go to Geoff, for all the time he spent during the year we were away, in typing out Sue's letters and forwarding copies to our family and friends; I'm enormously grateful to Janet and Martyn for their perseverance. I would not have finished writing this without their help and encouragement; to Anne, for trying to teach me to write English; and to Alan, for taking the raw material and turning it into this book.

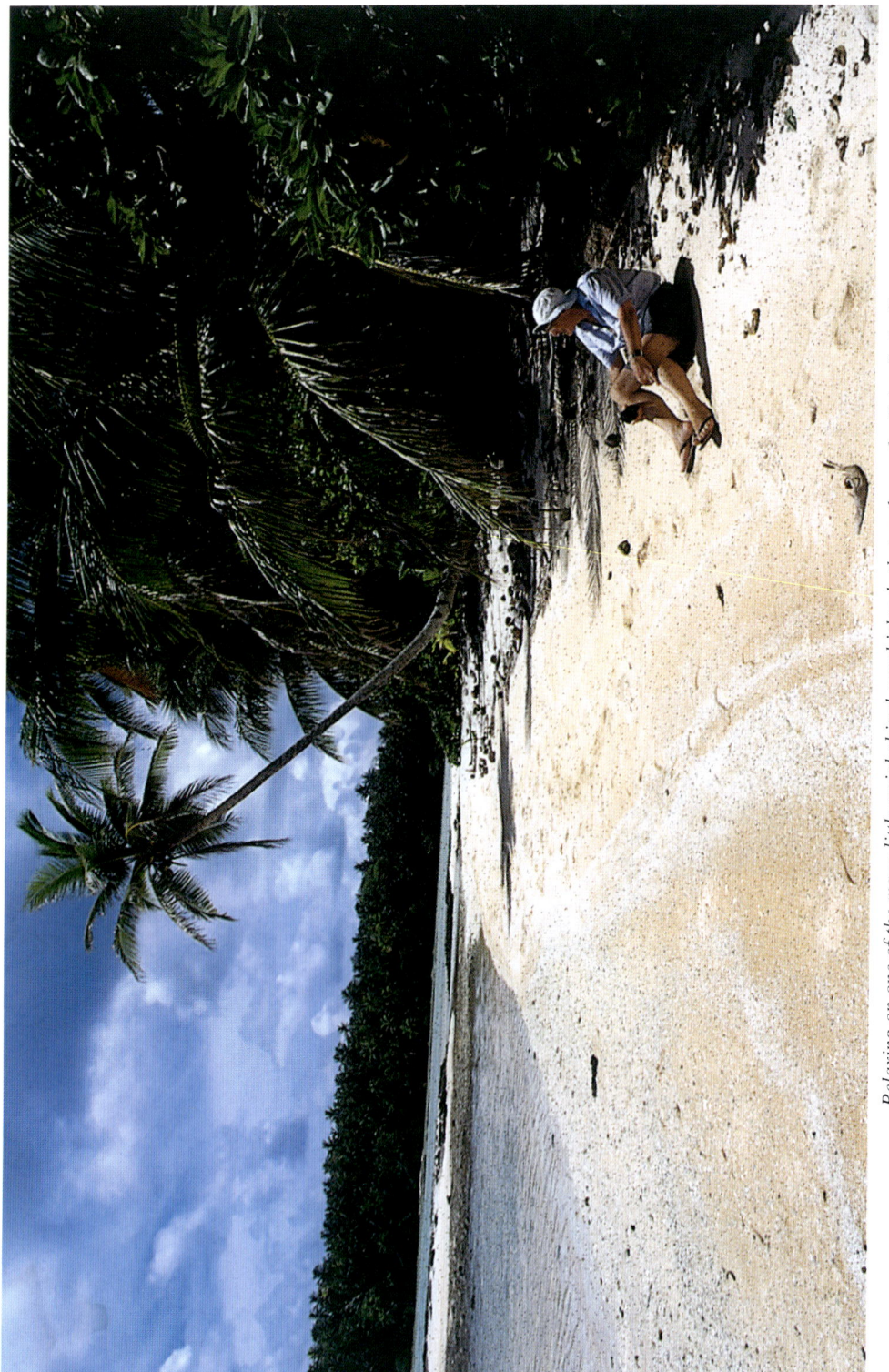

Relaxing on one of the many little uninhabited coral islands that make up the Fakaofo Atoll.

Where on Earth is Tokelau?

A doctor's experiences in the South Seas

Dr. Maxwell H. Heller

© Dr. Maxwell H. Heller 2005

ISBN 0-901100-58-7

Dr. Maxwell H. Heller asserts the moral right to be identified
as author of this work.

All rights reserved.
No reproduction without permission.

Typeset in Times New Roman
Printed and bound in Great Britain
by J.W. Northend, Sheffield
email: ks@northend.co.uk

Contents

A Series of Beginnings …	9
A Jump into the Unknown	15
Welcome to the South Pacific	19
The Doctor's House (or 'An Englishman's house is his goldfish bowl')	21
Life on a South Pacific Atoll	23
The Intrusion of 'Politics'	26
Christmas at 9° South	29
Trouble at Mill!	31
The wonderful, generous, infuriating people of Fakaofo…	34
From Doctor to Pathologist	51
Bolt from the Blue	51
Making the Best of Things	56
In the Doldrums	62
A Ceremonial Occasion	68
Ministering to the Sick	72
An Outbreak of Female Emancipation!	91
The Arrival of the Boat – And Farewell to Tokelau!	96
Back to Samoa	98
A Visit to New Zealand and Tonga…	100
Looking for Work (or Wheels within Wheels)	101
The Island of Savaii	105
Doctor in Residence (Samoan style)	107
Time for a Break	111
Crises in Casualty…	114
A Foreign Invasion	118
All Good, Clean, Healthy Fun	120
The Highs and the Lows	125
More Emergencies – medical and otherwise	128
An End in Sight	131
On a Wing and a Prayer	147

Foreword

A year in the life of an elderly medical doctor and his wife

This is the story of one couple's journey to the South Pacific and of their life on a tiny atoll. It relates their attempts to help the people of the atoll and to make sense of the customs and restrictions which ruled their lives. It is the story of an isolated hospital and the daily problems of maintaining it with little outside support.

Above all it is the story of the clash between a traditional society and the pressures exerted upon it by the modern world.

The islanders had taken to heart all the worst aspects of western society but had overlooked many of its better mores. We were happy to sell them tinned fish, although the seas around were teeming with fresh fish. We sold them vast quantities of sugar and forced them to live with the dental consequences. The incidence of heart troubles and diabetes was going up like a rocket, ever since we had encouraged them to adopt a western way of life and a western diet.

In trying to combat these ills as best he could, Dr. Heller was forced to confront both prejudice and downright lying. As he and his wife gradually lost faith in those in authority, so they gained the increasing trust of the local population. In the end they had to make the difficult choice between their need to escape from the duplicity and deceit of 'the system' and their commitment to serve the ordinary people, who were pleading for them to stay.

Having made up their minds, the couple continued to face new challenges and, despite all the difficulties, to build new friendships and attract new supporters. This is the story of a year in the South Pacific; one which shows what can be achieved with courage, determination and the support of a loving wife.

Maxwell Heller was born in Yorkshire in 1923. He was awarded a scholarship to the Royal College of Surgeons in Dublin, where he gained qualifications in obstetrics and surgery. His long medical career encompassed the fields of dermatology, general practice and anaesthetics and he finally retired from the N.H.S. in 1990. It is at that point that this book begins.

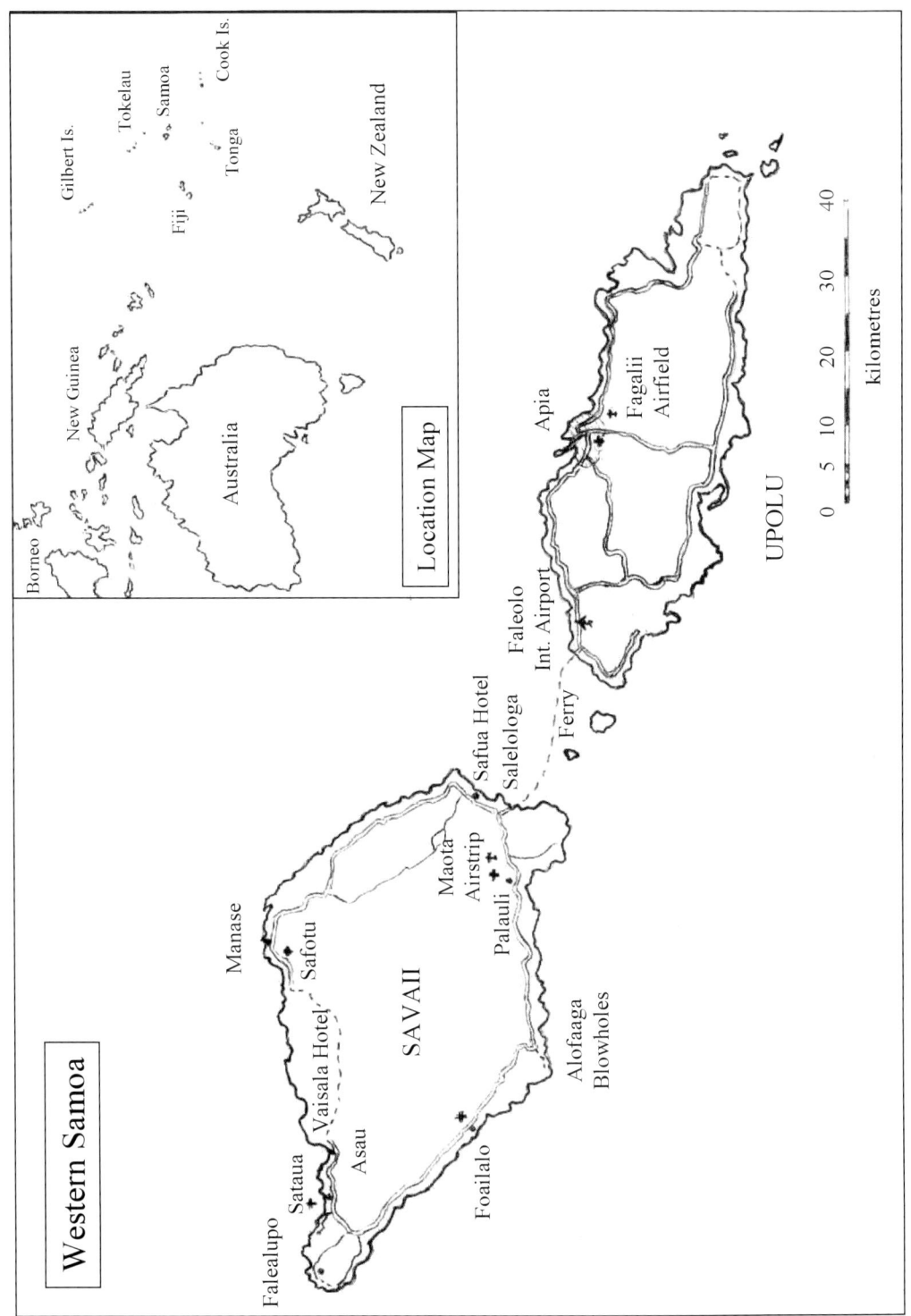

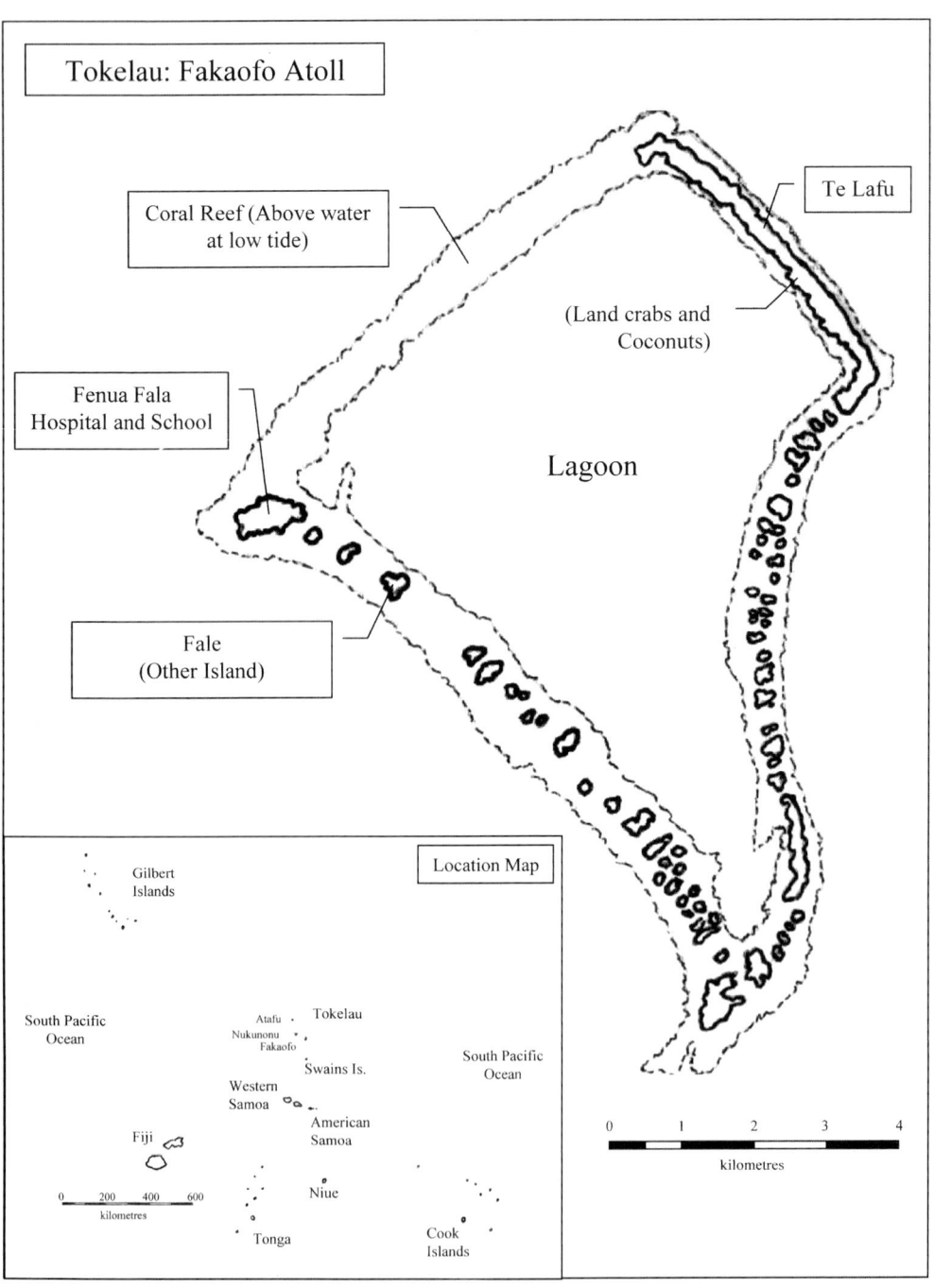

A Series of Beginnings

I think that everyone must have a secret dream; I know that I had. Many years ago I had read a book about Samoa written by Margaret Mead. There was my dream   **Samoa.**

After I retired in January 1990 on a very modest National Health pension, Sue, my energetic and ever-loving wife, said to me one day, "How do you fancy a trip round the world?" "Is the Pope a Catholic?" I asked. "How do we do it?"

To my mind, my pension was too small for that sort of escapade, but Sue had obviously been giving the idea some considerable thought. "How about using the Y.M.C.A. and Y.H.A.?" At this time I had already begun to think that my time was beginning to run out, but it was obvious that Sue had different ideas for me. "What about putting packs on our backs?" "You must be bonkers," I said. However, Sue started tramping the travel agents. To help us on our way, I went to work for a medical deputising agency to earn money.

After a number of false starts, Sue found a travel agency owned by a young woman called Judith, who, as the ideas were explained to her, became as enthusiastic as Sue. Sue has that effect on people.

As the old adage goes, 'In the beginning our eyes were bigger than our bellies'. Slowly the two of them whittled the journey down to a financially acceptable proposition. We could spend about four months going around the world and seeing most of the places that we both wanted to see.

The trip would encompass 10 countries, five chosen by me and five chosen by Sue, and it would be within the budget that Sue had decided we could afford. She had virtually every day priced out; so much for our bed, so much for food, so much for side trips and so much for pocket money.

Sue's work was fantastic. If only I could keep up with her. At the time I was 65 years old, came from a very short lived family and had recently been diagnosed by cardiologists in London as having triple vascular disease of the heart and that surgery was not advised: it would be a waste of time. I hope that those cardiologists live to read this story.

One wet and windy morning a friend drove Sue and me down to our local bus station and deposited the two of us, plus our large backpacks, onto the pavement to catch the London bus. We were ready to start the first stage of our round the world trip. There we stood, shivering in the cold and the wet, waiting for the bus to take us down to the airport. Were we out of our minds? Would we ever manage a fraction of what we had planned? Well, we did – we did it all – and much, much more.

It was whilst we were in Fiji, having a swim, that we met up with an Australian hat floating on the water. Underneath the hat was a very laid-back bearded Australian. He introduced himself as Steve and, after a few beers, we discovered that he was the chap in charge of the environment in Western Samoa. Over a meal that evening, after he had discovered that we were going to Samoa, he gave us a firm invitation to visit and stay with him. He even gave us clear instructions as to how we were to find him. "Just walk out of the airport, stop the first car and give the driver my card. He will bring you down to my office." It was hard to believe, and certainly I did not believe it at the time. But everything happened just as he said it would.

As we were shown into his office, he just looked up and said, "You are a day out." He was right of course. We had forgotten about crossing the International Date Line. This, I might add, caused me many problems when using my digital watch. It's much easier to carry an ordinary watch. Anyway, after his greeting, he just ordered a car from the Pool, and asked the driver to take us up to his (Steve's) bungalow. He gave the driver a bunch of keys, and said. "The beds are made up, show them where everything is, I will give you a ring when I'm ready to come home." Again, everything was as he said. The bungalow was large and the beds were made up, and better still, from Sue's point of view, there was an empty wardrobe and a nice clean bathroom with hot water.

After a cup of tea and a wash-and-brush-up, we almost felt human after the flight. The telephone rang; it was Steve telling us to get ready. "Go outside and stop the first vehicle that comes near and ask him to take you to 'The Love Nest'." Although we didn't realise it at the time, life around Steve was never going to be dull.

Have you ever thought of standing in the middle of the road in a foreign country and stopping an absolute stranger's car? We had not, not until then. But Sue did it. And once again, everyone was so nice; Steve's name seemed to be known by everyone we met.

The Love Nest turned out to be a type of pub, inhabited by at least one member of every nationality under the sun. We rapidly learned that they all belonged to some or other overseas aid organisation. We settled in comfortably. About 10 p.m. someone shouted, "How about Chinky Charley for food?"

About 20 of us piled into various types of vehicles and off we all went to Chinky Charley. I don't remember whether it was good or bad; all that I wanted was sleep but I do remember that on the way home Steve said. "Can you pack a small bag for the morning? We are going sailing with some friends at 6 o'clock." Remember, we had just flown in from Fiji. This was our introduction to the South Pacific and to what were called the Hash Harriers.

The Harriers were a group of people who were on loan to the various governments of the South Pacific. Some were teachers, some ecologists, some power cable engineers; some were communication experts, and all were people who might be useful to an emerging country. The group used to meet weekly to go for a run, followed by a big family barbecue. It was just a method of keeping in touch with each other and of knowing what was going on in various parts of the country and the South Pacific. We had been brought into their fold and made most welcome by them.

At six in the morning we were on our way down to the dockside. There, standing out in the bay, was what looked like a 40-foot sailing yacht and, from the sounds coming ashore, it was clear that a party had already started on board. An inflatable dinghy was powering its way towards where we stood on the quayside. No introductions were needed. Everyone seemed to know us. "Find a spot to settle down on. We have drink: beer, wine, vodka and there may be some food somewhere." It was now about seven in the morning.

We found enough beer to sink a battleship, but only one small bag of food. (The Aussies have their own priorities.) It was a perfect day. With about 12 of us on board we set out to sail around the coast of Samoa. Sue and I drank vodka and coconut juice; no one else seemed to like it. The captain knew where we were going, but he had no charts to help him find his way into the coral-shielded bay. The owners of this superb yacht had come to Samoa in the hope that they could start up a business, taking people out on trips around the islands of Samoa. This was their first chance to see how the boat behaved in the local currents. The journey should, we were told, take about six hours. By the time it got to early afternoon we still didn't seem to be any the nearer, and we were getting just a little hungry. The food was handed out (a sandwich each was the ration) and more drinks. By late afternoon we were becoming just a little concerned; we could all see the cove we were making for, but not making any headway towards it. The captain wouldn't start the engine and waste money on fuel, but the current was against us, so we were going nowhere fast. At 10 o'clock that night the boat dropped anchor just outside the reef and we were then landed by inflatable. *That* was an interesting experience.

Sue and I climbed into the rubber dinghy, followed by Steve. He seemed to know the drill. The little outboard was started and we powered up to the reef. The engine was throttled right back and there we lay. The captain grinned at our puzzled looks. Suddenly he shouted to Steve, "Now!" and to us, "Hang on!" He and Steve swung the outboard engine out of the water and sat and pointed for us to look. Racing towards us came the biggest wave that I had ever seen. We held on for dear life. The boat was picked up by the wave and lifted clean over the reef and into the little bay.

The whole village was there at the water's edge to greet us and help us out of the boat. They knew our names, greeting us as though we were old friends. The boat made four or five trips before we were all ashore, by which time it was after midnight. From the villagers we learned that they had been watching our boat tacking backwards and forwards all afternoon. The trip should have taken six hours, but, due to the lack of a good wind and no charts, it had taken 16 hours.

The food had been cooked and was ready, and had been for many hours, but the villagers had not eaten. We were to be their guests. Not even the children had been allowed to eat.

But first came the speeches.

This was our introduction to 'the speeches'. Everywhere we went, speeches started the meal, except when the church had the floor. It was an art form, and people took it all very seriously. Anyway it all went very well, and we eventually had food, and it was gorgeous.

The outside washing and toilet facilities had been demonstrated to us. The water came straight off the mountainside through bamboo pipes. We were very proudly shown their toilet bowl, and the pail for flushing it down. Toilet paper was the individual's own concern. Fortunately Steve had warned us about this need. Where it all went was not really obvious at that time of the day, but we could certainly smell its presence and proximity.

Whilst we were being shown their mod. cons, the women of the village had been doing the washing up and clearing the floor area of the communal *fale* (hut) and laying down rush mats and sheets, one sheet for each of us. Because I was the eldest, I had quite a bevy of girls attending to me. In fact, it was quite embarrassing; especially as poor Sue was more or less left to cope for herself. This was my first introduction to the Pacific attitude to the position of the female sex in their society. Sue was not impressed. She was even less impressed with the ladies fussing over me! Eventually, with a spray of mosquito repellent, we all settled down for a short sleep.

I slept well until about five, by which time others were already up. There was a mad scramble to taste the delights of the village shower and toilet. But the villagers were all so friendly and helpful. A good breakfast of fish, a stroll around the village and then back to our boat. One of the villagers decided to come with us. I believe that he wanted to visit someone or other in Apia. He also guided us through the reef. The journey back was uneventful, and with the wind and waves in our favour we returned in six hours. This trip around the Island of Upolu, the main island of Western Samoa, was our introduction to the Samoan people and their way of life!

The following day Steve took us up to the volcanic peaks to meet an Australian couple. He explained that they had left their own ranch in Australia, where they raised thoroughbred cattle. They had given it all up and put a manager in to run the ranch for two years, in order to teach the Samoans how to improve the breeding of their puny cattle into something like Australian beef. They were a wonderful couple. We stayed with them for some days. Their house was so high up in the hills that it was above the cloud line. Our clothing was damp most of the day. Also staying with them were three American teenage girls, who were supposed to be doing a project for their school back in the U.S.A. We never did find out exactly what this project was, but they were enjoying themselves.

The Aussie couple were not enjoying themselves. As fast as they managed to raise what they considered a reasonably bred animal, some member of the government would take it for barbecue testing, this being much more important, and definitely of benefit to the government. Dawn and her husband were becoming disillusioned and we were having our eyes opened to the realities of life in Samoa.

Dawn suggested we go for a drive down the side of the defunct volcano to the sea. There was one of the most beautiful beaches that I had ever seen, there right at the base of the cone. It was the classic Pacific picture postcard, and it was for real.

After a few days, Steve drove back up for us and we had to say our goodbyes. What had Steve got in store for us this time? His next suggestion came as a surprise, even to us. We had thought that we were getting used to his ways. "I have been thinking about a friend of mine on Savaii (which is the second island that makes up Samoa). I think that you should go and meet him. In fact, I rang him this morning. Pack a bag and get on the first plane tomorrow, I can drive you to our other airfield." I did notice that he didn't say air*port*. So, the following day, at about five in the morning, Steve drove us to Fagalii Airfield. It was about the size of an average football pitch. There were some pigs and chickens running around one end and some children playing football at the other.

We were weighed in on some scales under an awning, and we purchased our tickets in a shed, which doubled as ticket office and toilet.

The gentleman in front of us was larger than Sue and me put together. What sort of plane would it be? We knew that they had two planes for this inter-island run, but what sort? We soon found out.

A twin engine Cessna approached the field, and I can only describe its landing as 'one minute it was in the air; the next minute it had just plopped down on the grass and there it was in front of us'. The 6 o'clock plane had arrived. But it was not for us; by the time its cargo had been loaded and the very stout Samoan had been squeezed and pummelled into his seat, there was barely enough room for the pilot. No room for us. Thank God! We were informed, most apologetically, that we would have to wait. For what? "Next plane come soon." Meanwhile the plane with the very large gentleman and his many packages seemed to stagger into the air, rather than fly into the 'wide blue yonder'.

Shortly we heard another engine, the footballers scattered, the pigs ran for cover, and another similar plane arrived and pulled up, very nearly in front of us. A youngish pilot jumped out, strode towards us and shouted. "Any more for the skylark?" My faith in these small flying machines revived immediately. The pilot lifted his machine off the grass in about the space of two handkerchiefs.

The landing strip on Savaii seemed to be only the size of a single handkerchief, and that a lady's size. The New Zealand pilots really can fly these small Cessnas into incredibly small airfields.

Awaiting us at Maota Airstrip on the Island of Savaii was Warren Joplin, Steve's friend, and he was to become a good friend to us. He was a retired petroleum geologist, who had worked everywhere, north, south, east and west. He had found Savaii, Western Samoa, and made it his resting place and home. So well had he integrated into the Samoan lifestyle, that he helped many children from the village with their school fees. (In Samoa, all parents have to pay towards the cost of their children's education.) Then he had gone into a business, living in a Samoan style hotel, running a tour company and taking people around the island of Savaii. The hotel was owned by a Samoan lady, Moelagi Jackson. Her English name was the consequence of her marriage to an Englishman, who had died at an early age after suffering a massive heart attack. She now owned and ran the Safua Hotel, at the eastern end of Savaii.

Warren's name was known around the universities and better tourist agencies in that part of the world for his local knowledge, which was encyclopaedic.

Among the places that he took us to see was the Star Pyramid, a step pyramid which he had cleared out of the forest and cleaned. Then there was the Virgin's Grave, which had a delightful story attached to it.

A sprightly young man was chasing one of the village's young virgins. He was intent on stealing her virginity and she, rather than loose her most prized possession, threw herself off the cliffs. She was allowed to be buried in the church ground, in hallowed ground. Some time later, the local volcano erupted and lava poured down the hillside. Although the church was destroyed, the lava swept around her grave and stopped. The grave was saved, and also part of the village.

On yet another excursion, we visited the blowholes, which were spectacular.

The hospital at Palauli was the high spot for me. The nurse, who introduced herself as the matron, seemed to be the only trained person around. She said she had been trained in Canada. By the end of the afternoon she had found out all about us. She then asked if I knew what the piece of machinery was in the corner of her office. Apparently it had been sent by someone who had visited a few years earlier. They had thought it would be useful. It turned out to be an anaesthetic machine. "Would you stay and train someone to use it?" she asked. Unfortunately we couldn't, but we promised that, if it were possible for us to return, then we would come back to Savaii. There had been no doctor there for a few years. All around the island were small wooden hospitals, with just one or two nurses to take care of the people. With about 50,000 people on Savaii, they had a big problem.

We did not realise it at the time, but our trip to Savaii had marked another beginning.

Upon our return to Apia, Steve asked us, "As you are retired, would you consider coming back? They really need you. Come back and we will see if we can get some funding for you."

After we had returned home to the U.K., we heard nothing from Steve for some months. And although we tried to telephone both the hospital and Steve, we could not even get a connection. We had exhausted all efforts to obtain some funding from either this country or Europe. Everyone applauded our desire to help, but there was no money available.

In desperation we attended a meeting at one of our universities, a meeting sponsored by Voluntary Service Overseas. What a waste of time it turned out to be. First of all, they needed a signed contract for two years. Then I was informed that I was too old. And lastly, did I know how much it would cost to send me overseas? We both gasped when they quoted a figure of over £40,000. When I asked them to explain this figure, in view of what it had cost us, they explained it away by saying, "I would have to be watched over." "Watched over by another doctor?" I asked. "Oh, no. It could even possibly be me," replied our young interviewer. "Are you a doctor?" I asked. The answer was No. After this, he went on to explain that the staff and headquarters were very expensive. Sue and I did not wait to say goodbye. The meeting had made one thing very clear: if anything were to be done, it would have to be done by ourselves alone.

As I mentioned earlier, Sue and I had both returned to work whilst waiting to hear from anyone. Then after Christmas we heard that devastating hurricanes had swept over the South Pacific. The hospitals had been pretty well destroyed; the villages and crops had gone; communications, poor at the best of times, had been lost; Steve's work had been obliterated.

However, we kept on working. They must need us now more than ever, and the money that we were earning would be essential.

One day there was a letter for us, it was from Samoa, from Steve. He had a new job. He was now with the Tokelauan government, but still working for the environment. Were we free? Could we come out? The Tokelauan people needed us desperately. We had never ever heard of Tokelau, so out came the maps. Steve said that it consisted of a number of islands in the South Pacific, but, look as we might, we just couldn't find them. We purchased a good atlas, and there, above Samoa, three small dots indicated the atolls of Tokelau. We now knew where it was, but, try as we might, we could find no information about the people, or the islands. This sounded as if it could be the adventure of a lifetime. With no further ado, Sue started organising things. Eventually we even managed to speak to Steve on the telephone, and this marked another beginning.

The Consultants in our local hospital were wonderful, even showing me how to extract teeth, something missing from my previous medical training. They even presented me with a case full of old dental instruments.

A drug company and local chemists gave me a case full of out-of-date, but still usable, antibiotics and 40,000 aspirins.

One of the few things we *had* managed to find out was that Tokelau was a dependency of New Zealand and Air New Zealand generously offered to carry our excess baggage free of charge, as soon as they heard where we were going, and why we were going there. We were grateful also to Tony Doyle at Gatwick Airport and to Phil Rawlins, Cargo Manager at Air New Zealand, for all their help.

What more would we require for a 12 month stay on an island, about which we could find no information? Everything in our local library was outdated by 20 or 30 years and Steve had sent us only the most romantic view of things. "Just come. You will love it. Life is a dream, and the sunsets are wonderful." And so we set off.

In my 70th year, with a full life behind me, a new life was about to begin.

A Jump into the Unknown

Early on the morning of 24th September 1993 one of our daughters drove us – instruments, drugs and enough luggage to last for 12 months, down to Gatwick Airport to start the long journey to the other side of the world.

I am not certain if this was the flight where they upgraded us. Anyway, the flight was the usual boring, eating, guzzling time out. I don't know about you, but when I was younger I seemed to be able to sleep anywhere, but as I grew older, my ability to fall asleep on planes seemed to disappear. Stomach too full, boredom in full flight, nothing to do but disagree with my digital watch. We eventually learned how to cope with them. Just ignore them; you will eventually end up somewhere at some time or other. There was one occasion when we had two Saturdays and two Sundays in the same week. But that was all in the future.

All good things have to come to an end, and we eventually arrived at Samoa's International Airport; their one and only airport. We were met, thank heavens, by Steve and a very bonny looking Samoan lass. His introduction was rather confusing and somewhat disjointed. Or maybe it was we who were confused and tired, having been in the air for about 35 hours. We had flown from London to Los Angeles, to Hawaii, where we had a five-hour wait, and then on to Samoa.

The bungalow where Steve had lived in 1991, and where we had stayed, had gone in the hurricane; Steve was now living with Ava (we had eventually sussed this out) in her home, where we were going to stay.

Ava was a lecturer at the Samoan Teacher Training College. They both made us feel very welcome, but we were oh, so tired. However, there was a group of friends waiting, and food and talk. Fortunately Ava soon realised that we were asleep on our feet, flying on auto, and she sent us off to bed. Before drifting into sleep, Sue and I agreed, "It's good that they have found each other. They are right."

It took all of two days before we were back to normal. A couple of days later, Steve took us down to what was called The Office for Tokelauan Affairs. He introduced us vaguely to a few people, and then we were invited to follow another gentleman into what turned out to be a committee meeting. We were even invited to participate in the meeting, very strange. No questions concerning my work; in fact, no mention of my work at all. It was much later that we found out that the members of the meeting were under the impression that we were just interested spectators. They had all presumed that we were just curious and friendly visitors. No one had informed them that their new doctor had arrived and was there waiting to present his credentials and start work.

This was our first introduction to the world where the left hand would not let the right hand know what it knew or was doing. For if the right did know what the left was doing, the one would be as wise as the other and would be given an advantage, if you see what I mean? Later, their familiarity with this form of reasoning produced the most astounding reactions, such as when I started to lecture to the nursing staff, and they realised that I was actually trying to give them real information and an understanding of medicine. Other local doctors had offered them nothing.

The right hand must not know what the left hand knew, otherwise everyone would know.

It was some days later that we were introduced to a Dr. Liutta, the Director of Medicine for

Tokelau, and, in due course, to the other members of the governing body for the islands.

There seemed to be some hitch in the transport arrangements. The boat was delayed. This of course did happen from time to time. In the meantime, would I mind taking over the duties of resident doctor to the Tokelauan people who were living in and around Apia, the capital city of Samoa? In fact, it was the only real town in Samoa.

We were eventually offered a small bungalow on the outskirts of Apia, and were informed that a vehicle would pick me up each day between 8 and 10 o'clock in the morning. This occasionally did occur, when they remembered. If I was not there in the office, then the patients were seen by a 'nursing sister', who seemed to prescribe a coloured pill to every patient, a different coloured pill for each day. She had not actually killed anyone yet, at least to my knowledge. As I discovered that the pills were supplied to the office by a local chemist in packets, and were then sold to the patients in ones and twos, it seemed to me that, although they might not do much good, they were not going to do a great deal of harm. If any real medical problem presented itself in the office when I was not there, then the patient was sent up to the Samoan National Hospital, just up the road. That was staffed by a mixture of local and volunteer doctors from around the world. Most of the local doctors had received their training in either Fiji or New Zealand. The patients were charged, and were given a bill. This was then presented to the Tokelauan Office, which reimbursed the patient.

Meanwhile Sue and I were reading everything that we could lay our hands on relating to the Tokelauan Atolls. It all made for upsetting and depressing reading and it did not take a great deal of analysis to figure out that, medically speaking, the atolls were in a mess.

By their own accounts; on one atoll the doctor was an alcoholic; on another, the doctor was a Nigerian female who had been trained in Moscow, (I am not certain that she was actually trained as a doctor, because she had been under the impression that she was going out to the atolls to set up birth control clinics); and on a third atoll they had an elderly retired doctor. They did not want to talk about him, but we will, later in the story.

Time passed. Through Steve and Ava we were introduced to most of the volunteer crowd and to their amusements. Also, of course, through Ava, we met many Samoan people. It was all very pleasant.

We had arrived in September and already October had gone. Story followed story as to why there was no boat available. One day the newspaper reported that the reason the boat was not available was because it had hit something and the hole in the boat had been filled with a tree trunk! The next week the story was that its engine had developed some fatal illness, and had had to be sent off to some far distant place for repair. Actually most of the stories had some truth, but the real problem was that money was required up-front for the repairs. There was no money to put up-front. Therefore there were no repairs to the engine.

Eventually we heard another story. They had lost the crew!!

The atolls had an inter-atoll boat, which was licenced for those routes only. However, the licensing authority was in New Zealand, so they could do whatever they wished, especially as the atolls were a N.Z. dependency. This is exactly what happened. They were about to alter the licence of the inter-atoll boat, the Tutolu. It so happened that we had been advised, by all and sundry, not to travel on the Tutolu, no matter what happens.

Early in November, with just a few hours notice, we were informed that the Tutolu was coming in. "Get ready!"

Before leaving, I had a brief meeting with the Medical Director. He informed me that the hospital, the staff and all things concerning medicine on the Atoll of Fakaofo were being placed in my hands. By this time I felt that I was developing a good working relationship with him. He intimated that he intended that I should do all the things relating to the practice of medicine, leaving him free to write reports to the various Pacific organisations, and to attend conferences. He saw no reason why the arrangement should not work well.

Everything seemed clear. A sealed envelope was thrust into my hands; a few words of encouragement and off he went. Off too went Sue and I. When I eventually had time to remember to read the contents of my sealed orders, I wondered what sort of a magician I would have to be to satisfy all the requests. What sort of an idiot was I to try to carry out such an assignment?

We still had no information concerning living conditions on the Atoll of Faka, as it was to become known to us. Steve took us into Apia and we purchased some spices, flour, dried milk, tea, coffee, a few tins of fruit and a number of large white containers with good fitting lids, to keep all our food in. We also needed plates, cups and cutlery, along with a couple of saucepans and a very small gas cooker with an equally small gas bottle. It was beginning to be clear that Sue's Girl Guiding days of many years before would now be put to the test. All Steve would say was, "You will love it. The atoll is wonderful, the setting sun just needs to be seen to be believed."

Up until the last moment before getting aboard, well-wishers were still begging us not to go. "Wait for the big boat." But both Sue and I thought that we had waited long enough. It was time to get on with some real work.

The Tutolu, the boat in which we were to travel, turned out to be about 45 feet in length and of catamaran design, the passenger section being built across the two floats. It seemed to be a solidly built all-steel boat. However, no life-saving equipment was visible. The rear portion of the deck seemed to be full of chest freezers, which were steadily being filled with what looked like frozen meats. Small live pigs in boxes were being fastened to the deck rails. There was no plate to indicate how many passengers the boat could safely carry. Steve was chatting to all and sundry. Suddenly loud voices were heard. It was the captain ordering a man off the boat and the man was refusing to go. The altercation went on for several minutes before the captain finally said, "If you are not off this boat in two minutes, I shall switch off and close everything down." Believe it or not, this did the trick; the man jumped off the boat on to the quayside, still shouting back. But now, rather like at home, I thought, a police car was just drawing up and the man hurriedly got lost in the crowd.

What was it all about? The man wanted to go home to Tokelau, but would not accept that he had to purchase a ticket to travel on the boat.

Now it was time to go onboard and see what the sleeping arrangements were. The captain took us to our cabin. There were only two of them, one on either side of the boat. The one which we were to use was the captain's, and contained two single berths. The other one had just a single berth. Next to it was a toilet compartment. The rest of the covered portion of the boat was fitted out with rows of four-seater benches. Don't forget that the boat was really intended for inter-island travel, rather than deep-water ocean routes.

As the lines were being cast off, Steve on the quay side kissed Ava, who had also come down to see us off, threw a back pack onto the boat; and jumped onto the boat himself. "I'm coming with you," he gasped.

When Steve had recovered his breath, he explained that the Director of Medical Services had a paper that needed writing, and he thought that Steve and I could write it for him on the journey from Samoa to the Tokelauan Atolls. However, Steve fell ill as the boat was leaving the harbour, and he did not manage to stagger up from his bunk until we sighted our Atoll of Fakaofo. Nothing was written by either of us.

There was space for about 35 people on board, some sat on seats and some rolled up in sleeping mats or blankets and filling the available deck space. It was going to be an interesting crossing.

The captain had a helper for this voyage. Apparently to fulfil Board of Trade requirements, this elderly gentleman would, whenever he got the urge, disappear down into the bowels of the boat and spend some time there. He was presumably looking to make certain that the engines had not been stolen since he last looked, there being nothing else for him to do down there. The boat had twin engines and they just ran and ran.

Once we got out of the harbour and into deep water, Sue and I took ourselves off to look around the boat properly. Apart from the bodies everywhere, on the small rear deck we found a few faces that we had known from the Tokelauan Offices. One of them, a male nursing assistant by the name of Henry, explained to us that it was his duty to take all the frozen food out of the freezers and replace it with defrosted food, as there was insufficient freezer space for all the food which was being taken back. He had to repeat this process regularly until we landed. (Steve had never mentioned that there was any food problem!).

We then went off to pay our respects to the captain. What a great guy he turned out to be. He was a New Zealander, about 40 years of age. He was on his second marriage, his first wife having 'played the field', while he was busy with his sheep farm. He had sold off everything moveable and sellable in their home and had then gone back to sea and taken this job with the Tokelau Authority. He had met up with a New-Zealand-educated Tokelauan girl, who had herself made an unfortunate earlier marriage to a Samoan fellow. Both of them, John and Neta, were already divorced, when they subsequently met and married. They had set up home in Tokelau, which was her home patch and that of her family. John was now busy building a new and expanded home for Neta and the two children from her previous marriage. Everyone was happy.

In our opinion, the boat was a little beauty. She handled like a lady, even when we hit rough weather. We could only assume that it was the relatively small size of the vessel, in relation to the usual ship, which had caused such apprehension to the people on Samoa. Part way across to Fakaofo we called in at a small island called Swains; it had a beautiful weather-safe bay. We were to land supplies for the family who owned the island and lived on it. It was a sort of a *quid pro quo* arrangement. Our small inflatable, having taken supplies in to them, returned with a load of fresh lobsters, ready cooked. Whilst the lobsters were being cracked open, Sue and a few other hardy bodies dropped off the rear of the boat and had a swim. It was a welcome break, and the crustaceans were equally welcome. We had so far had nothing to eat but a few biscuits. The sight of the small galley and all the large insects crawling around the work surfaces had put an end to any thoughts of serving food from there.

The rest of the trip was equally good. Most of the passengers never moved from their sleeping mats. Steve never moved out of our bunk, apart from the swim, and Sue and I spent our time up in the small control cabin with John. He was happy explaining everything about the boat, even down to the system of navigation that he had installed. It even had automated satellite navigation. Brilliant! You did not even need to steer the boat, although Sue insisted on being allowed to man the wheel.

Our captain had a lovely story, with which he regaled us. It concerned a medical emergency… and Swains Island. A boat had set off from the mainland to pick up the patient. The boat had got lost and it took two planes to search and find it.

He followed this story with another, though I think that he must have had his tongue in his cheek this time. A boat got lost in fog off the coast of Samoa. It sent out a distress signal. When the boat was found, it was lying just offshore opposite the quayside.

On the third day, at about six in the morning, John said, "There it is, on the horizon, Tokelau."

Welcome to the South Pacific

"That small speck of sand is Fakaofo, your new home, your atoll, and for your information, it is about 900 miles south of the Equator. You will be on the first atoll and there are two others, both 60 miles apart, Nukunono being the nearer, then Atafu."

Landing was no easy business, John dropped anchor about 300 yards offshore on the seaward side of the reef. It looked as though a shallow passage had been blasted through the reef. Sure enough, a flat-bottomed boat was driven through this gap. On the shore there was quite a large gathering of people. They were separated into two groups; on one side vividly dressed women; on the other, the menfolk standing apart. In front of them all were two men, one tall and well built and the other, roly-poly. They were obviously the Dignitaries, or so we presumed. And so it turned out.

We stumbled ashore, and this was no easy task, for we had acquired our sea legs and seemed to have left our ordinary legs behind in Samoa.

There was no mistaking the friendliness of the greeting and welcome. Everyone wanted to help us up out of the landing barge. My legs seemed to want to be somewhere else. Certainly the land and the quayside seemed to be going in different directions, and I hadn't had a drink. As Sue and I shuffled forwards, the people pressed us on all sides and garlands of flowers were thrust upon us. We were led off the tiny quay, with much hand shaking. The two men who had stood in front eventually grasped my hands, and saluted me with much '*taileleia*' and '*feiloaiga*'. I guessed that this must be a welcome… I hoped.

We were led off down the quayside to what looked like a large building but had no walls, the roof being supported by tree trunks and the flooring being made of concrete covered with large mats. These large, loose mats were made of grass or leaves, woven into brilliant patterns.

Two white plastic chairs were placed at one end of the floor and Sue and I were led to them. Evidently these were seats of honour, as there were no seats for anyone else. This was clearly the Meeting House, and, equally obviously, there were to be speeches. The building rapidly filled with males, and I quickly realised that these appeared to be the Elders only. Outside the Meeting House were the women, children and younger men, sitting or standing around. It was on this first day that I learnt that the Tokelauans love making speeches. It was my greatest impression. As the day dragged on, I wondered if this was one of the remnants of the earlier Germanic influence, for they, the Germans, had at one time ruled the roost out here. There was still considerable old German tradition knocking around. This we had discovered in Samoa. There was plenty of evidence of old German family names and the remnants of the old style of German cooking. Also, of course there was the language. Until the Germans arrived, there had been no written Samoan language. However, the German intellectuals soon systematised everything and gave the people their nominative, accusative, genitive and dative, which every self-respecting language has to have.

A white-haired stockily-built man, speaking reasonably good English, came over and introduced himself to us. He was Dr. Zona, the island's old and retired doctor and a man for whom I developed a great fondness (but more of this later).

It seemed as though the speeches would go on forever. I found it rather odd, that Dr. Zona was not asked to say anything. At last, after about an hour, stumps were drawn, tables were set up, and food was laid out. The young people standing at the side of the tables were waving very large leaves to keep the flying creatures off the food. We, the honoured guests, were led to the table first. Now I had seen what the Samoans did, so I kept firmly hold of Sue's hand and led her to the table and at the table firmly pushed her in front of me. I was well aware that I was being watched closely by everyone, particularly by the women. I quite firmly intended that they should know from the beginning what I thought and how I viewed my wife's position. I was careful in future, at whatever function we attended, to make sure that Sue was always marginally in front of me. I had seen the attitude to women in the South Pacific and it was not to my liking.

One other thing we noticed was that the children always came last when food was being served. Not that it mattered on this occasion, as there was an abundance of food; in fact, far too much.

The plates were hand woven platters made out of leaves. We did our best, taking a little of everything, so that no individual could be offended by us not taking any of their particular cooking. Throughout the meal, women were constantly coming and plying us with extra morsels. It was an exhausting meal.

Sue, through an interpreter, spoke to a number of the women, enquiring which particular dish she had cooked, and how she had made it, etc. Meanwhile, the old doctor had moved around and sat on the floor at my side, acting as translator for those who wished to talk to me. Happily most people with a senior position on the atoll seemed to have some small amount of English.

Steve had disappeared as soon as we had set foot on land. We just wished he had given us a clue that this celebration was going to take place. We were very aware that, in our ignorance, we might make some enormous social blunder. About two hours later, it was indicated that the meal was over and our hosts were ready to take us to our transport, another boat, to complete the last stage of our journey. Our new home lay at the other end of the lagoon, and so, escorted by the entire local population, and covered in garlands, we slowly walked down to a small quay jutting out into the lagoon. Our luggage had been carried in a small boat from the Tutolu, which was anchored on the far side of the atoll, and brought to the jetty. We jumped into a larger boat (which we later discovered was the school bus!) and, accompanied by the headmen, sailed across the lagoon, with the English speakers excitedly pointing out the important landmarks with comments such as "The Catholics are buried over there" and "That is the wreck that poisons the fish." All good stuff!

It seemed that this atoll of Fakaofo consisted of two inhabited islands. After the hurricane, which had destroyed the hospital and the radio station, they had sent the younger people across to the island on which we were to live. A new school, a hospital and a radio shack had been built on it, as they considered it to be safer than the old island. There were several other islands on the atoll rim. One of them was given to newlyweds for their use after their wedding ceremony. No one could land on it without the Chief's permission. It had the best land crabs on the whole of the atoll, as they proudly informed us. At last our new home was in sight. A solidly built wooden bungalow-type building, with most of the upper part covered with glass louvered windows. It was about four feet above the level of the water, on a gently rising coral beach, and it was surrounded with coconut trees. Children galloped down to the jetty to greet us and to help carry our possessions into our home. Suddenly, as if by magic, we were alone. It was 9 o'clock in the morning and so much had happened already.

The Doctor's House
(or 'An Englishman's house is his goldfish bowl')

Up four steps to the front door, which opened directly into a largish lounge. It was probably about 20 feet square, and was furnished with a small kitchen table and four chairs. There were also two Ercol-type easy chairs and a similar three-seater sofa, fitted with thin foam cushions, which didn't make for comfort. On the floor was a native mat, which we later found had been made by the ladies of the village as a gift for us. The back door was more or less opposite the front door. Half way along the wall on the left was an opening into a corridor, which led to the other end of the house, into what was obviously the master bedroom. It was of a reasonable size, with louvred windows down to the floor on three sides. We immediately christened it the 'goldfish bowl'. On the left of the corridor between the lounge and our bedroom were firstly the kitchen and then another smaller bedroom, whilst on the right was a bathroom and toilet. The bathroom did not contain a bath, but more of these marvels later. First things first; we had to fix up the portable Chinese gas cooker that we had brought with us from Samoa. A cup of tea was needed. There were plenty of wall cupboards and a cursory inspection revealed that they were already inhabited. It was better to close them up quickly until we had had our drink.

Of course, all the directions for putting the cooker together were in Chinese and other Far Eastern languages. It took both of our mighty intellects to put all the bits and pieces together so that nothing was left over. It was a good Chinese puzzle, and it stopped Sue spending too much time looking in the cupboards. It did not appear that there had been a doctor living in this, the doctor's house, for a long time.

In Samoa we had purchased all the things we thought would be essential for our needs, even gas cylinders for the new Chinese double burner gas ring. However, it was only now that we realised just how Spartan our living conditions were going to be.

We would have added much more to our list had we known. Sue called me into the bathroom. She wanted to use the toilet. Would I please get rid of the other occupant? It was a rather large cockroach, about three inches in length, resting at the side of the pedestal.

Cockroaches can move fast when disturbed. So can Sue! It was an early sign of what was to come. We were going to spend a lot of our time battling against these creatures, and there were more of them than there were of us. It was guerrilla warfare from the beginning.

A further discovery was that the old, 50-gallon gasoline tank at the side of the toilet was not there for fun, nor for helping to put fires out. At this particular moment there was no running water. The flushing of the toilet was by personal arrangement only; hence the small can conveniently left beside the large tank of water. We had to learn in a hurry.

The beds had been made up European style, with hospital sheets, it being too hot for anything else. The wooden frames of the beds seemed to be afflicted with some form of livestock, so it was out with the insecticide spray and do as much damage as possible, then back to the kitchen. We had fortunately brought a number of plastic buckets with good sealing lids. This had been Steve's suggestion; he had been here before. These buckets would be used for storing some of our precious spices and foodstuffs, to prevent the insects getting to them first. There was a large chest freezer in one corner of the kitchen, which proved to have a large uncooked fish and a loaf of bread in it. However, as there was no electricity at the moment, we hurriedly closed the lid. Sue then boiled a saucepan, so that we could have a cup of tea. We hadn't purchased a kettle. After tea we explored the bathroom some more. There was an old sink with one tap, which looked promising, and there was a concrete shower stall with a large tap, such as is found on fire hydrants. The shower head had been made from the rose of a watering can, enterprising! Unfortunately none of these fixtures appeared to produce any flow of water.

In the kitchen beside the freezer was another sink unit. Once again it had one tap and once again it had no water. It was a good job that we had brought some bottled water, but the question was, how long could we make it last? In the corner opposite the freezer was a space for an electric cooker. I wondered where that had gone. The point was largely irrelevant, as there was no electricity. We later found that power was only available, when the generator in the middle of the island was switched on, for a few hours a day.

Whilst Sue decided to do a little unpacking, I went off to see what I could find out about the water and electricity supplies.

I knew that the hospital was located at the back of our bungalow, so I wandered in that direction and fortunately met up with Zona, the retired doctor. He gave me all the information I needed for the moment. The power would be switched on that evening at about 6 o'clock, especially in my honour. Normally the electricity came on twice a day; from 8.00 a.m. until about 11.00 a.m. and then from 7.00 p.m. until 10.00 p.m. at night. The water supply depended upon the power, and the old doctor took me to see this wonder.

The island had at one time had some shallow freshwater boreholes, fitted with hand pumps. But for one reason or another, the water had become tainted and could no longer be used. In any case, the little pumps were now rusted solid.

The hospital had been built on top of large concrete water tanks, even the doctor's house had been built on top of a tank.

"Why do we have no water in the bungalow?" I enquired. The reply surprised me. It seemed that there was no outlet at the bottom of the tank, only an overflow pipe at the top.

Where did the water come from? Rainwater, which fell on to the corrugated roofs of the hospital and of our bungalow, drained into the guttering and then down the drainpipes, which were broken in many places, into the concrete tanks built under the walkway around the hospital. I thought it best not to tell Sue about this, or about our private, but unapproachable, swimming pool situated beneath our lounge floor. At least, not until later!

How did the water get from these tanks to us? Behind the hospital I could see an elevated platform of wood and bamboo. On top of this stood a 50-gallon tank. The doctor explained that this was connected by a pipe to a pump, which sucked the water out of the concrete tanks and pushed it up into the 50-gallon tank. Gravity and the good Lord did the rest. I was mystified. This did not explain why we had no water; at least, not until the doctor spelled it out for me. It seemed that the pump had been loaned to us by the school, our pump having been broken and then lost. Unfortunately, the builders, who were building the new church, had needed the pump to mix another batch of concrete. Their need for water was considered greater than anyone else's, but the pump would be returned soon!

It was time to go back and tell Sue all about our private swimming pool. She was suitably impressed.

Later that evening there was a knock at our door. It was a little boy who said, "Water on!" and then ran off. We both dashed to the kitchen. Who was going to be the first to try the water?

When we opened the tap, it looked as if something was trying to crawl out, but then a thick soup of sludge slowly oozed out, followed by a gush of dirty water. We spent the rest of the evening trying to decide whether it was even safe to get washed in this water.

When the electricity came on, we examined the contents of the freezer more carefully. In addition to the loaf of bread, there was what looked like a whole baby tuna fish. We used the last of our first bottle of water for a final drink and departed for bed. The length of cloth at the windows was not large enough to cover half of the louvres, so we just climbed into bed and decided to try to get up early in the morning, before anyone could walk around our goldfish bowl.

No wonder Steve had found it difficult to describe things to us, and had just enthused about the sunsets. Never mind the sunsets!

In the morning I went off to introduce myself to the hospital and staff, leaving Sue to deal with the small unimportant things, like cleaning out wardrobes and persuading the inhabitants to live somewhere else. She unpacked not only our clothing, but also the considerable quantity of livestock, which had hitched a ride with us from Samoa.

Life on a South Pacific Atoll

Dr. Zona was already in the hospital and he introduced me to the staff. With the exception of the Staff Nurse, or Matron, whom he called Tocina, he did not mention the names of any of the nurses or assistant nurses to whom he introduced me. It was clear that he considered them too insignificant to be mentioned. I was beginning to get the picture.

When I spoke to Tocina, she merely moved her eyebrows. This could mean either 'Yes', or 'No'. Later I found out that she could speak reasonable English, but I also discovered that I was not her favourite person. This became so obvious that I had to ask Zona what was wrong. His answer was short and sweet. "You."

Dr. Zona was going to help me settle into the medical routine. The letter that I had been given by the Medical Director, indicating the things that he wished me to do, was so long, that there were not enough hours in the day for me to complete it. Fortunately the old doctor indicated that he was willing and happy to see to the out-of-hospital things, like visiting the school. For this I was most grateful. I got the feeling that he and I were going to get on very well together, and so it turned out.

My routine duties were allocated as follows:

Day	Morning	Afternoon
Monday	Diabetic and Blood Pressure Clinics	General Clinic
Tuesday	Antenatal Clinic	General Clinic
Wednesday	8.00 a.m.-9.00 a.m. Diabetic and Blood Pressure Clinics. Then Home Visits.	Home Visits
Thursday	Open Clinic (Anything)	Open Clinic (Anything)
Friday	Open Clinic on the other island, across the lagoon.	

There was also quite a lot of out-of-hours work, as time meant nothing to the local people. There were many incidents of children falling and cutting themselves on the sharp coral (all the Tokelauan atolls were coral, and just four feet above sea level), as well as, to my surprise, a lot of asthma and lower respiratory tract infections.

It did not take me long to discover that the level of medical and nursing knowledge among the staff was minimal. What I had learned in Apia was that professional people did not hand over information or knowledge willingly. In fact, it was guarded most jealously. For the sake of the patients, I would have to do something about that very quickly.

Later in the day Sue and I walked around the island. It took us about an hour, including a couple of stops. The first was to share a drink of coconut juice with a family of whom we were to see a great deal; at least we were to see a lot of their youngest child, Soshe. The second stop was to accept a rest and a drink of beautiful clear, cool water. This family had built their own large concrete water tank, which had an entry port for cleaning it out. Theirs was the best water on the atoll and they offered to supply us with water whenever we ran short.

The water that came from the hospital tanks was not really fit to wash in, but we had no alternative. Somewhere I have a lovely photograph of Sue standing in the pouring rain, under the broken down-pipe of the bungalow, washing her hair, with her *lava lava* wrapped around her. As she said, it was cleaner than the water that came from the tap, even though the rain was still heavily salted.

The following day was very hot, with no breeze at all. Sue spent the morning washing, having first to boil some water. She then left the clothes to soak in one of our large bowls, before rinsing them and pegging them on the line at the back of the bungalow. The humidity was so high she didn't think they would dry in a month of Sundays.

In the afternoon one of the nurses arrived with some home-made doughnuts. I don't know how they managed to get them cooked. We stopped work and had coffee, with honey and doughnuts. Lovely! Only later did our enthusiasm begin to wane, when we were attacked with indigestion. We suspected the fat in the doughnuts.

Dr. Zona called to inform us that there was to be a party in a few days' time. It was to be a welcome party for us. We thought we had already had one, but were informed that that had been from the Elders. This party would be from the people. It seemed that any excuse was an excuse for a party.

Two days later we were asked to be ready by 5 p.m. to be taken across to the other island for the party. The hospital boat was to pick us up. At 6 p.m. we were still waiting for the boat. We had to get used to Tokelauan time and not European time. Finally at 7 p.m. the boat came for us.

There was much singing and dancing, I found it difficult, as some of the women kept wanting me to get up and dance with them. That is one thing I can't do, as I have two left feet! The music was wonderful, no instruments, just a rolled up sleeping mat hit with a stick, and an old empty biscuit tin to beat out the rhythm. They just sang their hearts out for us. It seems they have no written words or music. The songs are just handed down from generation to generation. Sitting cross-legged on the woven mats, we were given plates made of coconut leaves and filled with food. Neither of us was quite sure what some of it was. We did recognise cooked green banana, mashed breadfruit with little coconut milk, and taro. The rest was a mystery. But the taste was good.

At about 10.15 p.m. the Roman Catholic priest gave a speech of welcome. The gist of his speech was to ask us to stay forever, as the people needed us. He then went on to tell a joke in his broken English. He found his story so humorous, that his belly laughter would not allow him to finish it, so we couldn't understand a word. He then said prayers and wished us all goodnight. So it was back to the boat and a dark crossing of the lagoon; the boys all seemed to know their way through the coral reef, so we just relaxed and looked up at the stars. They were so wonderful and so very many more than we could ever hope to see at home. It was even difficult to pick out the Southern Cross in the brightness of the sky. I just wished we had a camera able to take a photograph of it.

The generator stayed on for us until we got to bed at 11.30 p.m.

A few days later an invitation came for us to attend a wedding, which was to take place that same morning. It was already 8 o'clock, so we hurriedly got ourselves ready and waited for the old doctor and his wife to take us over to the smaller island where the marriage was to take place. We waited and waited, eventually, at 9.45 a.m., we were collected, only to find that we were too late. The service was over and the bride and groom were already in procession round the village. It was unbelievable. The bride wore a long, very full, white wedding gown with headdress and veil, but on her feet she wore flip-flops. The groom had a dark suit, which was a few sizes too big, especially the trousers. They looked as if they should have been turned up by at least 12 inches. He wore a white long-sleeved shirt with a large tie. And he also wore flip-flops. I wondered if these clothes were kept for every wedding on the atoll, but I didn't like to ask the question. With the temperature around 120°F in the shade and humidity of 100%, they certainly seemed very overdressed.

After the walk-about we all moved into the Meeting House and once again we sat crossed legged on mats. We had been placed near to the bride and groom, a great honour, but in this society the doctor always had the pride of place, which I found very daunting. The food was unbelievable; pork bits, fish, bread, or should I say half a loaf, doughnuts, green bananas, taro and a semolina cake. (We had never had that before.) It was all served on banana leaves. The party went on until mid-afternoon, stopping now and then for speeches, but most of the time was taken up with dancing. Eventually every one lined up and in turn shook hands with bride and groom, giving them presents or money. We had not come prepared for this, so could only give our congratulations. I don't think they understood English, so even that wasn't easy for us. It was only a little later, upon reflection, that we realised the reason we didn't get to the service. The old doctor and his wife wouldn't go to the church, as they were Jehovah Witnesses. It was a pity; we would have liked to have gone.

In the course of time, I was introduced to Dr. Zona's daughter, Leki. She was the only properly trained nurse, and the only one who had the faintest idea concerning nursing. She had also received midwifery training, and one night she was, I am certain, determined to find out what I was capable of doing.

It must have been about two in the morning when we were awoken by a pounding on the door. It was our nurse aid, "Staff Nurse wants you," she said. When I got over to our operating theatre, I found that we had a patient almost ready to deliver. There were no apparent problems. "I thought that you might like to deliver this one," Leki said. I think she had a slight smile on her face as she said this. In fact, I am certain about it.

You see doctors over here in the South Pacific do not really get their hands dirty if they can help it. This I had already discovered. Nudging her aside I took over the delivery and then stitched up the small tear. After this, I cleaned the patient up. As I got up from the stool, I smiled at the nurse and said. "Satisfied Staff?" With hindsight, it seems that that moment was much more important than I realised at the time. Anyway, the assistant nurse handed the baby to the mother and there was some conversation between Staff Nurse and the patient in their own language. Then Staff said to me, "How you sound your name?" "Max," I replied. Then turning from the patient, she said to me, "Baby now called Max. OK?" It happened to be my birthday, the 24th November, and it was 3.30 a.m. A few days later, as we stood at the door looking out over the lagoon, we were surprised to see a group of people coming towards us and pushing a wheelbarrow. Balanced precariously in the barrow was an electric cooker. "This is for you," they told us and proceeded to install it in the empty corner of the kitchen. I don't know where it had come from, but it was certainly going to make life easier than the little gas burner we had been using.

The days went by and Sue had done her best with our living quarters. Cleaning the house took no time at all. We could look straight through the floorboards on to the coral beneath, so she just swept the sand and dirt through the floorboards. There was no need for a vacuum cleaner on this island. She then started coming round the hospital with me. The condition of the buildings appalled her. Filth was apparent everywhere. It was obvious that no maintenance had been done for years. The solar panels did not work and the sterilising was a farce. The nursing staff considered that steam leaking from the lid of the steriliser indicated that it was working well. The seal between the body and lid had completely perished.

The Intrusion of 'Politics'

Tocina was supposed to be in charge; she was called Sister; but she did nothing. She was, however, powerfully connected. In fact, it did not take us long to discover that everyone appeared to be closely related. You had to be careful how you talked about any patient. Also there was a very marked pecking order.

Sue started compiling a list of what needed doing to the buildings and then made an inventory of our stocks of drugs, as no one seemed to know what we really had. However, this caused some friction with Tocina, who considered that these matters were her responsibility, and it produced a violent outburst from her. She was quite right; they were her responsibility, but she had not dealt with them. In the end she demanded to know by what right we were there and who did I think I was. This rather mystified me. I thought that everyone had been informed who I was.

Over the next few weeks this question arose again and again, not only from Tocina, but also from another nurse, who worked mainly on her own on the other island, where we had originally landed. There was a hut there, which doubled as a dispensary and an outpatient clinic, and which I visited each Friday. The 'nurse' had revealed to me that she had received no training at all. She too asked me what I thought I was doing in Tokelau. I felt that it was time to sort this out. I endeavoured to set up a meeting with all members of the staff. But this came to nought. I tried again, without success. Then I thought of inviting the *Faipule*, the headman, and the *Pulenu'u*, the mayor. That did the trick. They all turned up for the meeting.

I started by asking the *Faipule* if he would say a prayer for us. (I was learning.) Then I explained why I had called the meeting. I had come well prepared. Firstly I handed the *Faipule* the document from the Medical Director. Then I showed him photocopies of my medical qualifications. I suggested that this would be a good time to allow me to see the qualifications of the other members of the staff, so that I too would know whom I was dealing with. This, I might add, sank like a stone. I went on to explain how Dr. Zona and I would help each other in endeavouring to complete the task set by the Medical Director. I also explained the role that my wife would be playing in the running of the hospital, as no one else seemed to be doing anything about the state of the buildings, or their cleanliness. Nor was I satisfied concerning the drug situation, and my wife would tackle this concern as a matter of urgent priority. I then asked if there were any problems or questions. Tocina immediately asked who I thought I was? By what authority did I think I was there in her hospital? I knew this had to come. I turned to the *Faipule* and asked him if my qualifications were satisfactory, and, if they were, would he please explain to Tocina and the rest of the staff, in their language, what the situation was, as she obviously did not understand anything that I had just said. To my astonishment he did exactly that. The next question came from the 'Sister' from the other island, who had no nursing qualifications at all. She asked the same thing again. Why was I there? It was obvious that I was up against something with which I had not bargained. Some of these people obviously did not want me on the island. There were then a few hectic minutes when everyone seemed to join in. Eventually the *Faipule*, whose name I subsequently learned to be Melli, silenced them all. Turning to me, he said. "They will await and obey your orders." Then, turning to the audience "Dr. Max is the doctor. Enough." This was followed by hand clapping from most of the staff. Over the following week we continued seeing patients and I continued to give talks to the nurses in the afternoons, whenever we had time,

I had been told that the 'big boat' was due from Samoa. If we needed drugs for the hospital, or personal things, we should contact the Tokelauan office so that they could be purchased before the boat left. Now that was a problem in itself. In order to contact Samoa, we needed the help of the radio operator, but although we went looking for him, we never managed to find him. It was a little like the post office: no one around, and being told, "He has gone fishing."

After combing the island several times, we eventually found our man, and Sue talked to the office about the drugs we needed. She then listed the things we needed for ourselves, such as powdered milk and flour. We needed a very large bag of mixed grain bread flour. She also requested Coca-Cola, as she had found that the coconut milk disagreed with her when consumed in large quantities. As that was often all we had to drink, the situation was becoming urgent.

The imminent arrival of the boat made us realise that we had to get our letters and Christmas cards written. It would be our only chance to send them to the U.K.

While Sue concentrated on these matters, I was spending another scorching hot day in the hospital, dealing with more stupid problems. It was time for inoculations and I had just been shown the vaccines. They had been kept in a refrigerator which had no power supply for most of the day and all of the night. The inside of the refrigerator may as well have been the inside of an oven. The heat was killing the vaccines in their boxes. Although we had explained to the staff the importance of keeping the vaccine containers cool, it was obvious that they only did this if they were being watched. When we checked the temperatures in the insulated boxes, in front of the staff, the thermometer registered over 100°F. I then read out to them the instructions printed in large letters on the vaccine containers, detailing recommended storage temperature. Tocina, our senior Staff Nurse, just looked blankly at us. The vaccines were in the box; what was the problem? The vaccines had been taken out of the refrigerator and placed in the insulated box as requested. The fact that the refrigerator had been off all night and the overnight temperature had been over 100° was, in her opinion, of no consequence. However, this comedy of errors did not end. We discovered that the vaccines, having been delivered by the boat on its three monthly run from Samoa, had then been most carefully taken home by our police officer, our one and only police officer, and he had then kept them beside his sleeping mat all night, for safety. He had then proudly delivered them to the hospital's non-working refrigerator the following evening. [Sue has just corrected me. She says that they were actually delivered by a small child, with kind regards from the policeman.]

The first task the following morning was to find the lads who looked after the hospital boat. That was a feat in itself. Whenever you needed these people, you could guarantee that they would have gone walkabout. It may only have been a very small island, but people seemed to vanish into thin air. Eventually we found them and got them to take us across the lagoon so that we could buy stamps for our letters and cards. We were in luck, and the post office was open. We saw our correspondence put into the mailbag, but had to wonder whether it would arrive in England safely.

Sue now decided that, as we had an oven she would try to bake some bread. "It's just a question of getting the timing right," she said. The bread had to be cooked before the generator was turned off, which was usually around late morning, but unfortunately no two days were the same. She got started the next morning, as soon as we were up, which most days tended to be around 6.30 a.m.

I left her to it and went to see who was waiting for me in the hospital. As usual there were one or two of the Elders patiently waiting to see me. A number of families living in Faka didn't have any electricity, so it was bed at sunset about 7.30 p.m. and up with the sunrise at 5.30 a.m.

By the time I arrived back home at the bungalow, Sue had finished the first batch of baking.

It wasn't too bad, but flat – what one might call a little 'solid'. However, eaten with a little cheese, it was a nice change from fish. At least the electricity had lasted, which wasn't the case with the following day's bake. All Sue said was that she should have started sooner, and it might just have been cooked in time. The only thing we could do was to give the uncooked bread to one of our neighbours to feed to his pigs.

Christmas at 9° South

Christmas was upon us, but we could hardly tell, except by looking at the calendar. This told us it was Christmas Eve, but with no shops, festive food, or Christmas rush for the last bits and pieces, it all seemed very strange. It was just another hot, humid day. We waited for the wind to come, just to get a breath of fresh air. We had an extraordinary number of people coming into the hospital with lower respiratory infections, so we were kept very busy. Most of the nursing staff had gone home for Christmas, so it looked as if we would have a busy time. The only festive note was the choir from the Roman Catholic Church. They came and sang in the hospital. It was a lovely reminder, even if we didn't understand the words. The hymn that brought a smile to our faces was sung to the tune of our National Anthem, which seemed so odd. I suppose it relates to the fact that our Queen is the head of state, both of New Zealand and of Tokelau. The atolls were handed over to New Zealand in the 1920s and most of the population seem to think that the Queen lives in New Zealand. I didn't like to enlighten them. I don't think they understood that England is situated on the other side of the world.

Sue spent most of the night watching over little Soshe. He was a regular attender at our clinics. He had been brought in, as usual, when his bronchitis was verging on broncho-pneumonia. This time he had also got a beautiful asthma attack going as well. It was amazing how many of the islanders suffered with asthma. Anyway, I thought that this time he really did not have much chance of surviving. Our sealed cylinders of oxygen turned out to be as empty as most promises made to us. It was the same with the 50-gallon drums of gasoline and diesel oil, so carefully shipped out from Apia; they invariably turned out to be somewhat lighter than expected: everyone has to live!

Sue spent most of the night trickling our precious oxygen into Soshe, and alternating this with at least two other types of our out-of-date life-saving drugs. By morning, Sue was exhausted, but Soshe had recovered enough to make his usual disgusting noises. We now had nine cases of broncho-pneumonia, all of them children, and most of them from the other inhabited island across the lagoon. Only one case had come from our village. I was beginning to suspect that the patients on the main island were not receiving the correct treatment, or not being treated early enough.

On a lighter note, we did manage a small Christmas pudding brought from home as one of our presents. Sue cooked it in one of the hospital stainless steel bowls. We also had a cake, and some presents, given to us before we left the U.K., on the understanding that we didn't open them until Christmas Day. We had a laugh at some of the presents, a small box of waterproof matches, a metal tin to set a fire in, a small sewing kit, different coloured beads (to barter with?) and a small plastic bottle to send a note home to England! We also had a few Christmas cards and a tape of Christmas music to play on our miniature recorder. It was a welcome change. We were given some chicken drumsticks by John, the captain of the boat which had brought us to the island, so we cooked them with curry powder and rice, a very different Christmas lunch. We spent most of the day back and forth to the hospital, as the nurses were off for Christmas. As anticipated, the next few days proved to be busy and we were very tired by the time the nurses returned. One had gone to the top atoll to see her mother and her eldest child, the child being brought up by its grandmother, as she had remarried. It seemed to be the local custom to move children around between grandparents, aunts, and even friends who couldn't themselves conceive. Sometimes the children themselves would wish to stay with other people. That was the South Pacific way of life. In this respect, our observations supported those of Margaret Mead, made all those years earlier in Samoa.

Before we knew it, it was New Year's Day. Christmas had been so different; I don't think we shall ever experience anything quite like it again. Sue was told that we were the first British people to live and work on Tokelau since the missionaries came in the 1850s.

One evening I noticed a little boy running out of the hospital grounds holding what looked like a tin mug. I wondered what it contained and could only assume that it must be medicine. Sue had made good progress on the ordering and storage of drugs, but now it was time to start trying to check on their usage. It was very difficult; Tocina just raised her eyebrows when I asked about the tin mugs which I kept seeing children carrying around the hospital. In the absence of any proper explanation, I decided that no medicines were to be given out except upon my instructions. Each patient had to be seen at the hospital; it was not as though we would be overwhelmed. The population of each atoll was only about 500 people.

We kept a careful watch on the comings and goings. It was usually a child, but occasionally an adult, who arrived at the hospital carrying a tin cup and asking for medicine. This only happened when I was not there. It seemed that Tocina would usually oblige. After all, she had been running the hospital for many years, and her attitude, in common with most of the nursing staff, was that it didn't matter what tablets were given to the patients, because, if it were God's will that they die, then they would die.

The same thing was happening on the other island. Tocina's friend, Gimaima, the so called Staff Nurse, who was not even a nurse, turned out to be even better connected than most of the others. We had met her husband and knew him as Eeoh. We assumed that this was his name. It sounded very much like a Tokelauan name. We were wrong. Gimaima was married to the Executive Officer. This was the E.O., which had confused us so much. Everyone simply called him Eeoh.

However, to get back to the point, it was clear that Tocina and Gimaima would dish out whichever tablets they fancied for that day.

By now, Soshe was recovering, and, better still, one of our elderly patients was also recovering. He had been brought over from the other island, lying on a door placed across a canoe and then paddled across. He had been suffering from a rather nasty attack of asthma, complicated by a raging dose of bronchitis, but was now well enough to be discharged from the hospital. As was usual the whole of his extended family had turned up. They had been looking after his daily needs, cooking his food, massaging his extremities, entertaining him and in general watching over him day and night. This meant that there were sleeping mats everywhere, not only his, but also those that had been brought in for the relatives who had been his working party, and who had been looking after all his needs. This of course was normal practice out here. Praise was showered upon us. I do not think that either he or his family had expected him to survive this particular episode. Anyway the praise was fulsome and would come to be very helpful to us later, as it turned out that he was one of the most respected of the Elders.

The Elders were those men over the age of 60, who were thought by their peers to be fit to join the group which virtually ran the atoll. At that moment I began to believe that someone was looking after us; the conviction would keep us feeling human for a little while longer.

The fish diet was beginning to get to me; I was starting to feel like a fish. Certainly the fish were beginning to swim to me in much greater numbers when I sat under water in the lagoon breathing through my snorkel. On some days Sue would find it impossible to swim in the lagoon, saying that the water was too hot for her. I thought it was wonderful. We had one spot at the end of the island where brightly-coloured fish could be seen swimming in and out of the coral.

Trouble at Mill!

In spite of all the fine talk at Christmas, Sue and I were still being faced with the same old problems. Tocina was up to her old tricks again. This time she had decided that, as she had not had any leave, she would now take it, all twelve weeks of it. The Staff Nurse, Gimaima, who was no Staff Nurse, but merely the E.O.'s wife, came to work in the morning complaining of headache, shivers and shakes, and a temperature. "Then off you go to bed," I said. "Our patients are all ill enough already." Later in the day I was asked by Leki, why Staff Nurse was busy scrubbing out the visitor's house and not in her bed or at work. I too wanted to know what was going on. Staff Nurse had implied that she was too ill to cope with her hospital duties. Sue and I set off to find out what it was all about. The door of the house was opened to show the woman and her husband on their knees scrubbing the floor; we just stood there looking in at them scrubbing away. When she did notice us, she stood up and closed the door in our faces. At this I finally blew my top. Opening the door I shouted at her "Enough! I'm suspending you from duty until further notice."

Little did I know that this would eventually have virtually international repercussions.

Since arriving on Tokelau, I seemed to have spent at least as much time repairing broken equipment as I had seeing patients. Someone seemed to have been busy with a hammer and chisel trying to get into such equipment as emergency theatre lights. There was one very smart-looking emergency mobile light, with what looked like a heavy weight to keep it upright. On closer inspection I realised that this imposing looking base was actually a container. When I eventually got it open, I discovered that it was an emergency lighting unit with two massive batteries and a charging unit. Now, alas, it was rotten and corroded. No one had bothered to explain to the staff what it was all about. Still, this was all par for the course. Equipment had just been dumped on them for no reason and with no explanation. I suppose that was how we came to have a complete set of rib spreaders for opening up a chest, but no apparatus for putting the patient to sleep before one experimented with the equipment.

At one of our meetings with the *Faipule*, he had informed us that he had obtained permission to have a health visitor, a woman who had actually been trained in New Zealand as a health visitor. And best of all, because she already had a part-time job for which she was being paid (no one could have two paid jobs), she was going to work for free. There was insufficient money in our budget to have been able to fund her otherwise. She was a very intelligent young lady. Her husband was also a fully paid-up member of the teaching profession, having obtained his degrees in New Zealand. This of course disqualified him from being given any form of employment here in Tokelau, his own country.

You may wonder; why then had he returned? He had no choice. His parents were getting older. Someone had to come back to look after them. That was the custom, and so they did.

Incidentally, Sue and I had obtained some insight into the appointment of teaching staff, when we had sat in on the interviews for the post of Minister of Education for Tokelau. The woman who got the job was the perfect committee person. To virtually every question her reply was, "This is a question which should be referred to a sub-committee."

When appointing a new headmaster for our island school, preference was given to a real pedagogue, who presented the committee with a bag full of cards stating that he had attended numerous conferences and study days and various certificates of accreditation. It all looked very impressive, compared with the other applicant's Ph.D. and B.Ed., just two certificates! It was no contest. It was clear who would get the appointment.

It was about 6 o'clock in the evening. Sue and I had just done a ward round. The coughing from the patients made it sound like an old-fashioned tuberculosis ward back home in U.K. Staff Nurse informed me that all temperatures were normal. I supposed that what she was really telling me was that no one has actually died!

On the way back to our bungalow, Sue and I light-heartedly discussed the possibility of our two so-called Staff Nurses falling ill with some incapacitating ailment, maybe even some terminal ailment. It had been that sort of a day.

It was time for a nightcap, a little rest and recreation... I wondered if I had any Vodka left?

For a change, we had had a quiet night, with no disturbances at all. Now it was 6 o'clock in the morning. The sun was already shining brilliantly and nearly all the children of the village were down at the water's edge having their morning wash. We had heard a few little giggles, so we knew that one or two of the children were trying to peek into our bedroom windows, just to see if we were still in bed. It was time to get up.

Just like at home, mums, aunts, and even grandparents, were struggling to get the children to stop doing whatever they were doing and get ready for school. As mentioned earlier, the school was now on our island, having been relocated from the other island after the original school buildings had been swept away by the hurricane.

The local pigs were also on the move. The children had great fun with the pigs, and the pigs did just as they (the pigs) wished. I had informed the villagers that the next pig found wandering through the hospital would go straight into the stew pot, then to soften the blow, I said, "and it's going into the bowls of the old people." There were big smiles at this, whether of relief, or because they didn't believe me, probably both.

Sue had been saying how she would love a salad or just a bowl of fruit. But, of course, we couldn't just jump into our car and pop down to the supermarket. For one thing, no car... and for another, no supermarket! We had a few trees in the grounds of the hospital and I had been told, "If you find any fruit, it is yours." There was a hand of small green bananas, which we were watching carefully, and also a tree with one or two pawpaws. By lunchtime Sue had decided to climb the small pawpaw tree and pick the one and only ripe fruit. She reached the branch but, as she picked the fruit, the thin branch snapped. Down she fell, flat on to her back on the coral. Fortunately she was only winded and, after a minute or so, was able to get up. Her only concern was whether I had caught the fruit before it hit the ground. "That," she said, "will be for tea tonight."

Sue continued checking the stores, still struggling to enforce a simple but effective control system. The room was so hot that we could only spend an hour or so in there each day. We now wished we had brought with us a thermometer capable of high readings: I would have loved to know the correct temperature.

Our supply of syringes seemed to have gone down rapidly. Who could have taken them? Suddenly I realised what had been happening. We had been using them! This time it was down to us. Our stock of antibiotic tablets had been very old, some of them being over five years beyond their 'sell by' date. We had been getting so little response from the patients to these drugs, that we had switched them to doses of injected antibiotics. These had been donations from places like Austria, Bulgaria, China and other exotic places. However, the results had been virtually miraculous compared with the oral doses.

There was one room at the side of the hospital, which appeared to contain just a lot of old junk. As Sue went rooting through it she found two sealed packages, one a box about eight feet long and a foot square, and the other a packing case about three feet square. They had clearly been sitting there for some considerable time. The long box was marked 'A present from Denmark' and contained a beautiful stretcher, made of wood, metal and canvas. This had been lying in the storeroom, while patients were having to be ferried across the lagoon, lying on a door put cross-ways on a boat. The other case was labelled 'From France' and contained a brand new steriliser, of the large pressure-cooker type. This had a metal seal instead of the usual soft rubber seal. This was very important, as in the tropical climate of Tokelau a rubber seal would perish very quickly, as had happened on the steriliser we had been using. There were other packages lying in the storeroom. On opening them, Sue discovered medicines, mostly out of date, and about 2,000 needles. There were a few syringes – but no glass ones. I would have to think about this problem later.

In the meantime, Sue, like a magician, had just waved in front of me a large, no, a very large, container of multivite tablets. They were, of course, out of date, like everything else, but still, we had them, multivite tablets. We would give them to all our elderly patients and the children. It couldn't do any harm, and might even let their sores heal that little bit more quickly. Until this time all that we had been able to do was to paint their sores with gentian violet, even though I knew that the use of this substance is frowned upon at home. I believe that someone, somewhere, has shown that if you paint an elephant from tusk to tail with gentian violet for long enough, it eventually develops skin cancer, or something equally horrible. Anyway gentian was all we had. The atolls were made of coral, the people were bare footed; the children were forever falling and cutting themselves and the flies were everywhere. A good thick coating of the gentian violet at least kept the flies off the cuts and abrasions. The more Sue looked into and behind various cupboards, the more she found. Her latest find had been another brand new set of rib spreaders, not that we had yet found any anaesthetics. We had, though, found a present from New Zealand, an ancient anaesthetic machine with a very modern attachment. The attachment was called a Fluotec and, believe it or not, it was manufactured only a few miles from where we lived back home in England. However, the empty gas cylinders, which we discovered in an outhouse behind the hospital, were of a design called Pin index. Each cylinder had three little holes which had to mate up with three little pins on the connector; each type of gas had a different position for the holes. Hence the gas cylinder could only be made to fit onto the correct gas inlet. Unfortunately the anaesthetic machine had been made to take a 'bull nosed fitting', a type of screw top connection. It should have been obvious to anyone but our Minister of Health that the one would not fit the other. But how was he to know? He rarely visited his own country. His home was in Samoa; his wife had her business in Samoa; his children were at school in Samoa. And so the story goes on. The Tokelauans live on the Tokelauan Atolls and their government lives in Western Samoa. It is much more pleasant to live in Western Samoa than on the atolls. That is their philosophy.

The wonderful, generous, infuriating people of Fakaofo

One day we were brought, not only a bonito, but also some parrot fish. The colours of these parrot fish were so beautiful that it was almost a shame to catch them. In fact, I often took the snorkel and go and sit out in the lagoon just to watch the fish. For Sue and me the fish diet was monotonous, but it was far better than the meat. That meat which did occasionally arrive on the island, seemed to be an unusual variety, specially reared and exported for the Pacific Islanders. It was virtually all fat. But it was the same with their home-reared pork, inches of fat and only a thin sliver of meat

Back to the fish again. Sue loved the parrot fish, and, whilst I admit that the taste was better than the bonito, I could not stand the many small bones; I preferred the bonito's large bones and firm muscles. It could be de-boned quite easily and if soaked in sufficient spices, could almost pass as a piece of meat.

The same result can be achieved with a small tuna, as follows:

Recipe.   Take one tuna (or bonito), skin it first, then fillet it by using your fingers to take off the flesh from both sides.

Tokelauans would now hang it out in the sun until it was well dried, and of course well covered in flies. (It was strange that there is not a lot of diarrhoea amongst the people.)

However, I put my fish into a covered container to marinade overnight with soya or coconut juice. The next day, cut the fish into strips and place it under the grill to cook slowly. It can now be kept in a sealed container for several weeks. It's good for a quick bite when you are peckish, too tired or just nothing else in the larder. I suppose it's like the American 'Jerky'.

Despite the quality of the fish, we craved some salad, or fruit. In the tropical heat, we didn't feel like eating much, but we did miss fresh food.

A few days later, we noticed that the tide seemed unusually high; it was breaking high over the reef and into the lagoon. There was a mad scramble by everyone to pull the boats up the beach and well out of reach of the water. The waves were now breaking over the concrete jetty. Our bungalow was only a little higher up, and normally the water in the lagoon would be three to four feet below the level of the jetty. As the whole atoll was only about four feet above sea level, we feared that it would be inundated, particularly when we had one of the sudden, brilliant rainstorms, so typical of the area. However, the danger passed and the tide subsided. Sue had not been wasting her time; she had taken advantage of the downpour to have a refreshing shower in the clean rain. She had also collected enough rainwater to give our dirty clothing a thorough wash. How she managed to keep us supplied with clean clothing every day was a mystery to me, especially as our supply tank had a habit of running dry just when water was required.

A major drain on our resources was indirectly caused by the patients themselves. For every patient, there were usually a number of relatives, all of whom had to be accommodated. They provided their own bedding, as well as clothing and pots and pans, but these all required washing, a procedure which consumed a large quantity of water. Therefore the high level tank would be liable to run dry at some time during the afternoon. This itself would not have been a problem, except that the generator was only switched on in the evening, so there was no power for the pump until then. And always lurking at the back of my mind was the realisation, as I had learned on that first evening on the island, that the pump feeding the tank really belonged to the school, which might decide to reclaim it at any time.

There were additional complications. The connections to the pump were comprised of many pieces of old inner tubing and were very susceptible to failure. On one occasion, the workers had been messing about all afternoon, trying to get some sort of a seal on the suction side of the pump. The high-level water tank was empty and the pump was sucking only air. It seemed to be difficult for them to think in an orderly fashion with regards to electro-mechanical things. They seemed incapable of starting at one end of the system and working through until the defect was located. The confusion was compounded by the enthusiastic advice and argumentation from all the bystanders.

I suddenly became aware that what they had been cutting up and using to make a seal was an Esmark (a three inch wide, rubber elastic bandage) from the operating theatre. "God help us," I thought, "if we need to apply a tourniquet to stop someone bleeding to death." This had always been one of my worst fears when watching the young children playing around the sterns of the boats, particularly while an outboard motor was being started; I was terrified. Here we were, at a hospital with no running water and possibly without even any tourniquets. I guessed that 'Florence' would have known what to do! I was not so sure that I did!

That night I went to sleep thinking about how to make repairs to the water pipes. I would have to try something tomorrow.

The next morning I woke up still thinking about water. As old Dr. Zona had told me, the lounge of our bungalow was actually built over a massive concrete water container, fed by a drainpipe from the roof of the house. It collected water very efficiently. There was only one thing wrong; someone had forgotten to put an outlet connection at the bottom of the tank. Therefore, if we wished to use the water, we would have to set up a pump and try to pump the water into one of the hospital water tanks. Unfortunately we did not have sufficient piping to allow us to try this, and so the water lay there, and we sat on top of it! The water in the deeper parts of the tank must have been as old as the bungalow. Our friend Steve had informed me that there actually had been a source of fresh water on the island, but it had become polluted, like so many other things out here in the South Pacific.

It was always as well to keep some boiled water in the freezer, although, even when boiled, it was sometimes too disgusting to drink. For those occasions I would ask the lads to bring some fresh coconuts every day, open them and chill the milk. Personally I enjoyed coconut milk with just about everything; heated up it made very acceptable tea, coffee, or cocoa; and I was very partial to it as a nightcap, mixed with vodka. My other luxury was a dash of rum with the coconut milk. Some times I needed it. Sue preferred her cup of chocolate with powdered milk. When we ran out of the milk, one of the nurses told us that there was a family selling tins of the powder. We asked her if she would obtain a tin for us, only to find that it was twice the price we would pay in Samoa. It was a good example of private enterprise; whenever the families had any spare cash, they would purchase extra tins of anything that they thought might be in demand before the arrival of the next boat; then they would sell it for twice the price.

By this time, we had been on the atoll for several months and I had become very friendly with old Doctor Zona. His was a rather rum story, which was particularly interesting in that it threw some light on the religious tensions on Tokelau.

As a young man he had been sent to Fiji to train as a doctor. Whilst there, he had become involved with the Jehovah's Witnesses, a religious group which held a different faith to that which prevailed on his home atoll. On returning to the island he had joined a small group of similar believers, and they had commenced holding prayer meetings in Zona's home.

Now there are basically only two religions on Tokelau. The original faith was established by missionaries from the London Missionary Society, (L.M.S.) in the mid-19th century. The story goes that, at a later date, some people, claiming to be teachers, asked for permission to set up a school on one of the other atolls. This they were allowed to do. However, it turned out that they were actually Roman Catholic missionaries. That is how there came to be two religions. One atoll was Catholic, the second, where the church had been established by the L.M.S., was Congregational and the third, that on which we lived, was a mixture of the two faiths, with Catholics being in the minority.

Dr. Zona and his little group of Jehovah's Witnesses had been discovered and had been banned from the atoll. It had only been in the recent past that he has been allowed back. He was still not really accepted and was treated rather shabbily, especially by his relative, Tocina.

Since arriving on the island, we had not seen much of our friend Steve, but he continued to be active. It was one of his responsibilities to look after the environment, but it was an uphill struggle all the time. His latest fight was in trying to get rid of the nice, friendly, communal, 'over-the-water' drop closets, which were located at the beach, just over the water in the lagoon. They were, of course, built in the nicest places. The people loved to sit and talk – and empty their bowels. However, this was also the favourite area for the children to swim and frolic and also for the pigs to congregate. It was amazing that the hospital was not swamped with cases of diarrhoea and vomiting. However, I have seen more cases of those ailments since I came back home to England than we ever saw on the islands. Steve's difficulty in tackling this problem was that, although the cement for the building of proper cesspits was reaching Tokelau, most of it was being used to build a monstrous new church on our island. But Steve persevered, despite the frustrations. He even tried to get the islanders to eat a healthier diet – like using brown flour and brown rice; like eating margarine instead of butter and taking less sugar. It was all to no avail. Boatloads of the nutritious and healthy products had been sent back to Apia, to be replaced with boatloads of tins of corned beef and fish. The corned beef appeared to be specially produced for the Pacific islanders; it was so full of scrag-ends and fat, that it would have been banned or rejected out of hand in any other part of the world. The islanders had developed a taste for tinned meat during the last war, and some bright boy had realised that here was a ready-made market for all the stuff which we threw away from our slaughterhouses. It was a great idea! And who, in his right mind, would have considered shipping tinned fish to a Pacific island, whose only natural products were fish and coconuts?

All this created yet another problem, where to dispose of all the empty tins? This was still unresolved at the time we left.

Tokelau must have had the biggest and fattest flies in the whole of the South Pacific and, when someone cut himself, flies would settle on the cut immediately. Nearly everything became infected. It was our custom to put any edible waste into a plastic container outside our back door, to be recycled to the pigs. However, sometimes the pigs got to it before we had a chance to get it to them! The mess and flies were incredible. They had to be seen to be believed, which was why Sue was busy videoing the black swarm of flies settled on the coral.

Since arriving at the island, Sue and I had been recording the different ailments which we had encountered. From this information, we tried to figure out the best and most economical drugs that were really necessary. Even so, we knew that our head office in Apia would have a heart attack when they saw our list. The trouble was that they seemed to be buying in small quantities from a local chemist's shop in Apia – never anything like the amounts we needed.

There was more to this than simple inefficiency. I had already learned that Tokelau had the authorisation to purchase necessities directly from New Zealand, under the auspices of the New Zealand government and at a large discount. In addition, no shipping costs were charged to the Tokelauans. There were only two drawbacks: firstly one had to have the foresight to place the order well in advance: secondly, and potentially fatally, the system allowed no opportunity for the little perks and back-handers, which were so essential to business in the South Pacific. The system was doomed from the start.

Accepting that any supplies we were to receive would have to come via Samoa, it would be necessary for me to book some radio time, so as to place an order with Apia. We had to ensure that we received the medications when the next boat arrived. Not that we knew which boat it would be, for there was a rumour going about that there might be a 'new boat' in the offing. The old one, you will recall, was suffering from a number of serious ailments, which to me, as a trained doctor, appeared terminal.

Rumour was the main source of information out on the islands. The girls in the radio room listened in to nearly everything which came over the airwaves, but reception was usually very poor, so the messages were often garbled. There was no telephone communication, the cables having been severed by the earth tremors many years before. There was, of course, the radio transmitter, but the operator was only on duty for a few hours each week, so rumour and gossip was the best that was available. This did not limit the discussion and speculation, which were the main topics of conversation, except for cricket, or *cricketi*, as it was called by the islanders. Their version was a wonderful game. The only way in which it resembled that played in the rest of the world was that there was a ball: there was a club that vaguely resembled a bat; and there were three stumps. As to the rules, your guess is as good as mine is. Any number of people could take part, and they did. If one side was dissatisfied with the result, then they simply demanded a replay on the following day. After all, there were no deadlines to be met. The fish would still be there in the sea, the breadfruit and the coconuts still there on the trees, and plenty of time for eating and drinking.

From time to time, the flow of gossip and chit-chat came in useful. One evening, at about 6 o'clock, Sue told me that she was just going to remove the petrol tank from the hospital motor-boat. She had heard whispers that two of the young lads, who helped out around the hospital, and chauffeured us around in the boat when we needed it, had been taking it out for midnight joy-rides. We wondered whether that was how the original outboard motor came to be damaged and then conveniently lost.

Shortly after the incident with the water pump, I was approached by Leki, our good Staff Nurse, or, should I say, our very good Staff Nurse, who presented me with a document and asked me what I thought of it. I was astonished. It was fantastic. The nurses had got together to set out a series of rules and regulations concerning the staff, detailing the way they should dress, their time-keeping and recommendations in respect of their hours of duty. There was also a list of staff responsibilities and even a note saying how they thought we should recruit young junior staff, by merit, rather than by blood relationships. In fact, the document contained all the ideas, which Sue and I had been trying to get Tocina to introduce. And here were the nurses offering it to me just like that. It just demonstrated to us that the younger people did understand what we were trying to do for them. It showed that they appreciated that the traditional ways, where everything depended upon a person's position in the pecking order, to whom they were related and how old they were, were not necessarily the best ways.

The problem with relatives was becoming acute. We had admitted a new patient, broncho-pneumonia, a classic case, right out of the textbook. However, he had so many relatives that we were running out of space. They had taken up the whole of one ward. It was beginning to look as though we were going to need a ward for each patient. Fortunately an injection of the Austrian penicillin appeared to have been effective, so it seemed we would be able to release him quite soon. While preparing the injection, I had noticed that we were very short of syringes; and the few glass ones were so dirty that I could not get them to look clean, even to the naked eye.

That afternoon I went over to have a chat with the *Faipule*. He was a nice person, as his name Melli would suggest. He told me that he had never wanted to be *Faipule*. The islanders had virtually forced him to accept the position. He had had little alternative but to accept the honour. Anyway, he wanted to know why I had suspended the Staff Nurse. I had come prepared for this very question, and handed him a paper on which I had typed out the various reasons:

1) Absenting herself from duty when she was supposed to be there, leading to complaints from patients
2) Being rude to patients
3) Refusing to see patients when it did not suit her
4) Adopting an irresponsible attitude to the patients. For example, playing cards when on duty and ignoring reasonable requests by patients to be seen
5) Giving out medicines in single doses, sometimes without even seeing the patient.

And finally in my opinion

6) Dereliction of duty, and ignorance of the very basic principals of medical knowledge or nursing practice.

I finished it all off with my own personal blast. I asked how she came to have received the title of Staff Nurse, when she had completed no formal nursing training. I did not add my own thought that marrying the Executive Officer was all that she had really needed.

The *Faipule* pondered this unwelcome complication to his life. As usual, it came down to money, as everything did, in the end. "If she is not working, who is to pay her?" He gave me to understand that no one had the authority to actually fire anyone. Only New Zealand had the power to do that, or, at least, that's what he said. Somehow I doubt it. I shrugged and told him that it was not my problem. I was simply there to run the hospital and see to the needs of the patients.

As the other island now had no resident nurse, I had asked Leki to go across and look after things until I could sort it out on a more permanent basis. Before she went, I gave the staff a talk on how to tell the difference between Cardiac Asthma and Bronchial Asthma. Later Leki told me that Dr. Zona, her father, had been very upset with her because she had not informed him about my lecture. I was becoming aware that my talks were becoming very popular. The staff were beginning to look forward to them. Zona came to our bungalow later, bringing a bottle of beer with him for us to share, whilst we talked about this and that, which gradually developed into a discussion on the afternoon talk. In future I would have to remember to invite him to my talks, although it was all pretty basic stuff.

Over supper that evening Sue and I were reminiscing. Before we had come to Tokelau and while we were still living in Apia with Steve and Ava, Steve had come home one afternoon and said, "I've got a good deal. Come to Niue with us. It's a good cheap deal." He said that he had been there several times before and 'knew people there'. (Where didn't he know people?) We didn't need much persuading, so… off we all flew. Sue and Ava chattered away as if they hadn't seen each other for weeks, while Steve was obviously waiting for a chance to speak to me very confidentially about something. When the opportunity arose, he whispered to me that he wanted to marry Ava and he thought that Niue would be the ideal place. "Would you be my best man?" he asked. He knew the local priest and the registrar, so he did not foresee any difficulties.

"How does Ava like the idea?" I asked. "Oh, I haven't asked her yet." That was Steve, full of the best intentions in the world, but prone to go off half-cocked. Sue and I had often talked about their relationship. They were so obviously right for each other and it would be a good match. "That's good," I said, and it was settled.

It was a beautiful island and, of course, Steve knew the hotelier involved in the promotion. The hotel itself turned out to be made up of a small group of Swedish-style chalets built about 40 feet from the edge of a vertical cliff. Trees surrounded each chalet, except for the view to the west. It really had to be seen to be believed. It was a picture and Steve really did know the owner, an expatriate Australian, and his Polynesian wife and children. There was also a restaurant bar and a small dance floor, situated next to the chalets. It was all most friendly. The New Zealand High Commissioner, who was also married to a Polynesian wife, used to drop in for a pre-prandial drink. It was all very pleasant and civilised. We settled in to our two chalets, or rather Sue and Ava did. Steve and I trotted off to hire a car for the following day. He had still not revealed to Ava what he had in mind.

The following morning, on the pretext of picking up the car, Steve and I went off into the tiny hamlet to have a chat with the priest and the registrar. The hire car had actually been delivered to us and left in the car park at the back of the restaurant, but Sue and Ava were unaware of that. In the space of an hour it was all sorted out; a special marriage licence had been purchased; a time had been set for the wedding, which was to take place the following day; the registrar and the reverend father had been briefed.

We collected the girls and had a good day driving around the island. Eventually Steve revealed his secret to Ava. He also showed us where he wanted the ceremony to take place. He had, on a previous visit, seen a beautiful fairytale grotto, about two hundred yards from the cliff edge. Ava was non-committal and we left them that night, talking it over.

The next morning dawned, as magnificent as ever. The sunrises were out of this world. By the time we had breakfasted, the wine was already in the refrigerator and the champagne was on show, waiting to go in the chiller. 12 o'clock came, and the couple sauntered down, to inform all and sundry that they were going for a walk. The wedding service was scheduled for 1 o'clock. There we were, the registrar, the priest and the guests; we all sat waiting. At half past one, in came the happy couple, but not as bride and groom. Ava had persuaded Steve that this sort of wedding was not what she wanted. She wanted a typical Samoan wedding. She realised that they did not have the money for a full-blown Samoan celebration and they were not going to throw themselves into debt, as many Samoans did. Therefore they had compromised. They would have a Samoan-style ceremony, but with a restricted wedding list: a mere 100 or so guests. But that was for the future. As we were all here, let us all have a nice time. We had the champagne and the wine; we could make it a day to remember, and that's what we did. Sue and I were beginning to learn the Polynesian way.

The liquid afternoon blended smoothly into a liquid evening. I vaguely remember being introduced to a gentleman, who we already knew was the New Zealand High Commissioner. He in turn introduced us to his very glamorous Polynesian wife. Food arrived, greatly appreciated after so much drinking. Then the evening's entertainment began.

The band was good. The audience appreciative, but many of them had been slaking their thirst even before we had arrived and they began to insist that they should be allowed to sing with the band. It was just like a boozy sing-song at home. We said our goodnights, and went off to our bed. Just before going to sleep I remembered another person to whom we had been introduced by Steve. She was the Minister of Health for Niue. She had asked us if we were free, as she had some vacant positions in the hospital that required filling. I remembered the look of amazement on her face when we explained that we were already committed to going to Tokelau. Looking back from where Sue and I now sat, reminiscing about our trip to Niue, it was easy to understand her reaction. Anyway, we had accepted her invitation to visit the hospital on the following day. It was a splendid little unit, with only two doctors, and one of them being only a volunteer from New Zealand, staying for just a few weeks. We ended the day by being taken to 'The Hotel', freshly repaired after the last hurricane. Someone had had a camcorder at the time, so had been able to record a video of part of the storm. The force of the wind was unbelievable; we were shown a boulder, about eight feet in diameter, which had been thrown up from the beach, some 100 feet below. If we were beginning to feel apprehensive, it was because we knew that Tokelau was only about four feet above sea level. What would such a storm do to a South Pacific atoll? Thinking about all this I dropped off to sleep.

Sue was having a difficult job in trying to motivate anyone to do anything to remedy the effect of years of neglect on our hospital building. But we were not alone; everything was in the same dilapidated condition. Even Apia, the capital of Western Samoa, looked like a studio set for a third rate western, with the odd modern building thrown in. Things were built and then left to deteriorate. Maintenance was a foreign idea and not really understood. The very concepts of conservation and good housekeeping were completely foreign to them, hence the decrepit state of the medical equipment and the parlous state of the buildings. The filthy state of the hospital was almost unbelievable. The toilets and the washing facilities were an absolute disgrace; the walls were covered with fungus of delicate shades of green and brown; the floors were like a skating rink, lubricated with slime and filth.

One of Sue's problems was that she was a woman, and this was a male dominated society. There was only one way to solve this problem, and Sue set about it with a will. She had to shame them into doing something for themselves. She set to work on the broken drainpipes. Quite a crowd came to see this little Palangi woman (she is only five foot nothing in height) up on a ladder repairing broken fall pipes with some discarded tin cans, a tin opener and some wire. She became quite expert at cutting the cans in a spiral so that she could join the two ends of a broken pipe together. In case I forget *Palangi* is the Polynesian term for any white person or European, though my dictionary spells it *Papalagi*. Sue's pleas over the radio to the Tokelauan government in Apia back in Samoa had at first been met with a warning "Don't rock the boat." However, the people here were now beginning to talk about 'their hospital'. Daylight was beginning to dawn on them. I sat the children on my knee when examining them, I visited the elderly and the infirm in their *fales*. They could see that we ate the same food that they ate. We were getting on famously with the people – especially with the children.

The next boat actually brought timber, piping, guttering and paint. Though admittedly, the bills of lading didn't match what was off-loaded to us. Still it was another victory of some sorts. Sue's magic with tin opener and old tin cans had won her a place in their hearts.

The grapevine began rustling again. There *was* to be a new boat, well at least, a new second- or third-hand one. It was to come from New Zealand. Actually, we often heard these rumours long before the authorities received the information. After all, our radio operator had nothing to do all day after his scheduled stint had finished. Nevertheless our best source was Neta, the Tokelauan wife of John, captain of the inter-atoll boat. This was the catamaran which had brought us from Samoa to Tokelau. The boat and captain were registered only for inter-atoll travel. However, when the situation required it, the registration was miraculously changed. We had become very good friends with John, Neta and their children. Now Neta was no ordinary Tokelauan. She had taken her education seriously and had achieved all she could on the atoll. She had eventually been sent to New Zealand, where she had trained to be a dental nurse. Being a dental nurse in the South Pacific is not the same thing as in a developed country. The dental nurse automatically becomes the dentist. That is how Neta arrived back on the atoll as its dentist,

John had fixed up a set of transmitters and receivers so that he and Neta could talk to each other in private, but she could also scan virtually the whole of the South Pacific airwaves. Nothing was hidden from them when they chose to listen in, which is why Neta was always our best source of news.

When the boat arrived this time, it deposited a load of what I call free-loaders, although that is not really fair; some of them were genuine do-gooders. We had been informed of their imminent arrival. There was a husband and wife team, together with their child. The man was only there for the ride, but his wife had an assignment to write a paper on the educational needs of the atolls. She was good, but not really necessary. Everyone already knew what the educational needs were, but the authorities insisted on hiring these 'experts' at exorbitant fees to write papers, which would not be read, but it did keep the experts off the streets. The responsible agency, known as S.P.R.E.P., or South Pacific regional-some-thing-or-other, hired these experts and, once they were on the agency list, they were in the honey pot. Certainly nothing was ever done as a result of their reports. A few meetings were held, resolutions were passed and further papers were written. It kept everyone happy, and the money flowed in and out.

It was at about that time that we became aware of much 'muttering in the undergrowth'. The local people were beginning to hear murmurs from the other atolls that they wished Sue and me to go and do for them what we were doing here on Fakaofo. Old Zona called in to ask if there is any truth in this rumour. He said that the people of Fakaofo did not want us to leave the atoll, although he knew that we would be welcomed on Nukunono. If necessary he, Dr. Zona, would be prepared to go in our place.

With all this rumbling in the background, life in the hospital went on much as before. I had again been awakened at four in the morning; this time for the admission of one of the Elders. He was in *status asthmaticus* and in a bad way. I had to use the last of my supply of intravenous hydrocortisone which was within the 'use by' date and then followed this up with a bottle which was out of date. It worked a treat! In my opinion, this whole 'sell-by date' thing is a load of cod's wallop.

The patients were wonderful. The relatives were wonderful. They now realised that we were trying to help them. It gave us a warm feeling when we got away with something which we had no right to expect. Saving the life of the Elder was one of those occasions. What is it that was written, 'If my right hand forgets its cunning, etc., etc.'?

By the following afternoon the old man was asking if he could have a little fish, raw fish. He was obviously improving rapidly. The people loved raw fish, especially when mixed with coconut juice. In fact, I was beginning to develop a taste for it myself.

Amongst the people who had arrived on the boat was a nursing Sister from the Tokelauan Office in Apia. She was a close friend of Tocina, who had already tried to take over the running of the hospital and we had angry words almost from the moment she stepped ashore. Anyway, as we were so short of staff, I asked her to come in to the hospital and help out. To my surprise, and that of everyone else, she came in for work. As usual, the cause of the trouble was poor communications. What the director had told me verbally was totally different to the written instructions, which he had given me at that last moment as we boarded the boat. His verbal directions were that I should be fully responsible for the running of the hospital and that I should assume authority for that. He had made no mention of work in the community or outside the hospital, aspects which were clearly detailed in his later communication, whereas the fact that he had delegated to me full authority over the hospital staff appeared to have slipped his mind. In fact, his written instructions were as follows:

DR MAX HELLER
VOLUNTEER – ENGLAND
WORK REFERENCE

Attend to the supervision of:

A. Outpatient Clinics
    i)   General
    ii) Diabetic and hypertension
    iii) Pre and postnatal clinics
    iv) Maternal and child health, pregnancy and family planning

B. Inpatient
    i)   Management and follow-up
    ii) Obstetrics and gynaecological cases
    iii) Referrals

C. Public Health
    i)   Maternal and child health programme and family planning
    ii) Immunisation programme
    iii) Health education
    iv) Village inspection with community reps
    v) Health programme
    vi) Epidemic and disease surveillance and reporting
    vii) Record of epidemiological data

D. Environment Programme
    i)   Waste management programme
    ii) Environment awareness
    iii) Vector control programme
    iv) Public safety

E. Training
    i)   On-the-job training for nurses
    ii) Staff seminars and workshops
    iii) Community groups – workshops and seminars

It turned out to be a good day, and an even better night, as I got a full six hours sleep. It is wonderful what a good night's sleep will do for you.

The next day we were able to discharge some of the babies, which freed up a little more space, so we were able to move the old boy out of our operating theatre and into a ward. He was doing very well and his new position gave him a good view. He loved it. I can still picture him, surrounded by his many relatives, with two little toddlers, barely able to stand, staggering down the ward, hand-in-hand. One stumbled and the other, trying to help him, grasped his friend's head in both hands and pulled him to his feet. Everyone laughed; it was a gorgeous scene.

We continued on our list of drug requirements. As we never received what we had ordered, we were forever making up new lists. I, or rather Sue, had discovered that we had over 1,000 tablets of a drug used for treating tuberculosis, even though to date we had not seen a single case of the disease on the atoll. There were two other things on the day's agenda. First, and most important, cricket! After that I was hoping to give a talk to the islanders on AIDS. I don't think they knew what it was! But the priority was the cricket, which, of course, would be accompanied by feasting and holidays all round. Zona would share the day's workload with me. I would go over to the other island for the morning's affray; then, when I came back to the hospital, Zona would go over for the afternoon. He loved the *cricketi*, and the singing and the wonderful wit that so enhanced the game. It had poured with rain from six until seven that morning, which was good, as it kept the dust down a little.

My thoughts kept coming back to water. We seemed to have used so much since Christmas. Although the pump was working well, the suction piping was in a pitiable state. Our wonderful handyman Lau, pronounced Pee-au, seemed to be able to scrounge bits of elastic from all over the place, I think that he had a secret horde somewhere, or maybe he had taken all the elastic bandages out of the hospital. He was probably right. The pump's need was greater than ours. Lau was one of nature's gentlemen. When you were busy, nothing was too difficult for him, and he would stay around all night, if necessary. He would just stretch out on one of the long forms in the outpatients department and drop off to sleep. He was so useful that we wished we could put him on staff. We informed everyone that, in the meantime, he should be treated as one of the staff. What a change we saw in him when we explained what we were trying to do. Status is everything, and our simple action worked wonders for his self-esteem.

Holidays, speechifying and food, they seem to be the main industry and the main products of the atolls.

Sue was getting very tired. She seemed to be picking up all sorts of minor ailments. I think the place was beginning to get to her and the rumours were not helping. There was a rumour that Dr. Liutta, the Medical Director, was coming over, that he had been instructed to come out to the islands and actually live there. And the wildest rumour of all was the suggestion that the whole government might be forced to come out and actually live in its own country! Sue had recently spent much of her time scrubbing and cleaning the wards, so that all would look good when the Director arrived. I was feeling tired for her.

Over the R.T., Dr. Liutta was making vague suggestions that we might move to another atoll and do for them what we were doing on Fakaofo. He also asked what I would think of one centralised hospital for the three atolls and what would we require for one centralised operating theatre. Although these approaches were in the strictest confidence, he must have known that the conversation could be overheard by anyone else listening in. It was therefore no surprise to me when, later in the day, Melli came over to see me. Would I consider staying on this atoll as a permanency, he enquired. "What do you mean?" I asked him. "Just stay with us." The Elders had asked him to speak to me. I explained to him that our air tickets would only allow us to stay for twelve months anyway, but he felt sure that the Elders would be able to sort this out, the atolls were after all a dependency of New Zealand and our tickets were with New Zealand airways. They were of the opinion that something could be sorted out.

It was very pleasant to hear this sort of thing. But could we really continue as we were? While the islanders on our atoll were obviously very happy with us, it seemed that those in official positions did not share this view, and we were the piggies in the middle.

That day we had a meeting with Mr. Liena, who was one of the people dropped off by the last boat. It seemed he was from the W.H.O. It was nice to listen to him. He said that they were aware of us and of our work, and were impressed with what they had heard from the local people. We decided to wait and see. It was encouraging to hear so much praise, nearly three hours of it, but would it actually result in any changes?

With all that talk, I had really developed an appetite during the afternoon. Unfortunately the best we had available was fish jerky; but at least it was filling.

We had just received a blade of pork, which was our share of meat from the village. We would have to think very carefully about how to cook it, as it was over fifty percent fat, considered a great delicacy by the islanders.

There was bad weather forecast, so I had to go out to drop the storm curtains. Whilst doing it, my attention was drawn to a strange shape on the shore. I would have sworn that it was a mythological creature, with white hair and staring eyes. Was that a tail protruding from under its cloak? I had to call Sue out to see it. She thought it was a turtle… but it turned out to be just a rock formation and a trick of the light.

Our usual problems were ever-present. We would go to bed thinking about them and of course they were still there when we awoke in the morning – the shortage of water, the faulty toilet in the hospital, which overnight had emptied the high level tank. We hoped that these problems would sort themselves out. Personally I was feeling awful, but not because of these practical difficulties. This was more physical. I had a throat like a piece of raw leather, accompanied by a bad attack of shivers and shakes. I knew that it couldn't be malaria, as we did not have that type of mosquito on Tokelau, at least, not yet! I struggled through most of the day, but then took to my bed. By the following morning I was feeling well enough to supervise what was going on in the hospital, but it was a considerable time before I was feeling back to 'my old self' again.

Sometimes we could lose sight of the difference between our background and that of the Pacific islanders. One day while examining a pregnant patient, I said to the nurse aid, "Come and listen to this." It was the sound of the foetal heart and of the uterine arteries. "It sounds like a steam train," I said. "What is a steam train?" she replied. For most of them, the world beyond Tokelau just didn't exist.

There was much talk concerning independence for Tokelau, which, from New Zealand's point of view, I could well understand. The atolls were a real financial drain on them. We heard that it was costing over 4,000,000 dollars a year to keep the Tokelauans afloat, and there were only 1,500 of them, distributed over the three atolls. However, the Elders are far too smart to fall into the independence trap. They can see how it has left Samoa; independent but bankrupt.

Clearly something would have to be done to improve nursing standards. I seemed to be getting more aggravation every day from the nurse who had come on the last boat from Samoa. I suspected that the Medical Director has sent her to find out what was happening on the island. Tocina and her friend Gimaima had been burning up the fax transmitter. These two women certainly did not like us. In fact they probably feared us. We were upsetting their cosy little set-up. They were a powerful duo and they had a lot to lose. It was obvious that they had been able to control Dr. Zona, but felt very aggrieved that they were now unable to have their own way.

Life on Tokelau did have its lighter moments. We sometimes heard amusing stories, such as that concerning the gentleman who was nominally the Financial Director for Tokelau. Of course, like all the prominent officials, he lived in Samoa, rather than out on the atolls. Accountants had been sent over from New Zealand to have a look at the books. When the Financial Director was eventually found, he was unable to produce any figures for the previous six months, nor did he have any books available. Sue and I were not altogether surprised. While we were still in Apia, we had been invited to dine with the Financial Director. He had picked us up in his new four-wheel-drive vehicle.

His house turned out to be only about ten minutes drive from where we were then living. It was set in the middle of an extensive banana plantation and with a large field at the back of the house. There were a number of cattle grazing in the field. He explained to me that the estate, for that is what it was, was just a small part of the property owned by his wife and himself in Samoa.

The house itself was not the usual timber building, but a modern solid shelled architect-designed bungalow. It had been built with a high and steeply pitched roof, beautifully cool. A small entrance area opened into a large lounge-cum-dining room, about 30 feet square. The furnishings included a grand piano, a very large television set, and an equally large radio and music centre. The dining area contained a large dining table, set with ten chairs. The kitchen, which was open-plan held a very large double-doored refrigerator. The house was beautiful and, as the Financial Director pointed out, it was very conveniently close to the golf course. He was pleased to show it all off to us and we were suitably impressed. Who wouldn't be? Sue and I could understand anyone's reluctance to leave this altogether delightful situation to go and live on a coral atoll.

After what we had seen, we were not surprised to learn of his difficulty in explaining the accounts. But we shouldn't be churlish; he had given us a lovely meal. Although he was eventually replaced, he did not get the boot. He was just moved sideways to an equally lucrative post. Everyone was related to one another, and no one fired a relative!

As fast as I managed to resolve one problem, I was faced with another. I wondered whether any vestige of our work would remain after we left. Or was I simply making things worse by showing them how things could be improved? The younger nursing staff were ready for change. They really needed it. As things were, they were not even *playing* at doctors and nurses. I would have to talk to the *Faipule* about all this. It was worrying me.

The younger nurses were really trying hard and they were asking questions all the time. That was wonderful. Suddenly they could see a future for themselves and for their hospital; not only that, the people talk quite boastfully about *their* hospital.

The arrival of the official visitors had generated not only rumours, but also many meetings, both open and clandestine. The airwaves had been busy and the inter-atoll boat has been going back and forth like a yo-yo. I was excluded from most of the meetings, but the *Faipule* had kept me well informed. The Elders were obviously enjoying themselves. There were so many opportunities for speeches. It was the aim of everyone to be a good speechmaker and that required the ability to speak for half a day before getting round to the nub of the matter. The speakers were egged on from all sides and they were applauded continuously. A good speech would be remembered, and, anyway, it was a good way of passing the day.

Meanwhile we were at the centre of our own little intrigues. The *Faipule* from the other two atolls had sent their minions to entreat us, and even to offer little bribes, to persuade us to go to their own atolls. However, we liked Fakaofo and we had, in any case, given our word to Melli.

To say that we liked our atoll is not to suggest that our life was idyllic. I had noticed that Sue had not been filling in her diary recently. When I asked her about it, she said, "I'm sick of all this argument and I'm tired out." It was a shame, after all the hard work she had done for them. To be honest, if we had not let our house for 12 months, I might even have thought of calling it a day and of leaving the islanders to their own devices. I felt so sorry for Sue. We had been offered work in Apia, but we no longer believed anything that we were told; even though it was apparently said in good faith! Sue continued to write her monthly letters home, but not with the same enthusiasm. They were sent off when, and if, the boat arrived from Samoa. At least we could now be reasonable sure that they would be posted. We had discovered that the office, where the postage stamps were kept, was run by the husband of one of the nurses. From her we learned that he only opened the office when the boat was about to leave on the return journey to Samoa. But why couldn't they have just told us that in the first place?

Sue had another disappointment. She had decided to bake some bread and needed to open the large sack of mixed grain flour, which had come on the last boat. To her horror, she found it crawling with weevils. She was advised to sieve it and use it. That was what the local women did all the time. It had to be cooked anyway. Sue couldn't bring herself to do that and it finished up being given away, supposedly to feed the pigs, although I imagine that it was a welcome addition to some other family's food supply!

The following day one of our boys turned up for work. He had gone A.W.O.L. on New Year's Eve. The spirits had overcome him. He still had the headache! Leaving him to his woes, I went to talk to Dr. Zona concerning contraception for the women on the atolls. His advice on the subject was ludicrously simple; why didn't I think of it before? "Just tell the men to *go fishing*," he said. The whole topic was not taken very seriously. As Dr. Zona said "The girl will marry whomever her parents tell her to, regardless of her having had a baby or two by other men." This was true, and it sounded all too familiar.

Whilst on Tokelau, I had time to re-read Margaret Mead's book on Samoa. Perhaps, at this point, it might be appropriate to describe the subject of her book and what impact it had had on the ethnological debate of the time. It may also clarify why I, as a young man, had been so influenced as to still have a yearning to visit the country more than 50 years later.

Margaret Mead was a young academic of 25 years of age, who had just finished her doctoral thesis when, in 1925, she was sent from America to carry out a study of the youth of Samoa. The purpose of the study was to resolve a dispute which had been raging in academic circles for the previous 15 years, namely: was a person's behaviour influenced more by his genetic inheritance than by his environmental circumstances? This was summed up at the time in the phrase, 'Nature or Nurture?' Most biologists favoured the genetic theory, but by the mid-1920s, the anthropologists, in favour of the cultural argument, were in the ascendancy. Margaret Mead, under her tutor Professor Frank Boas, was of the latter school of thought.

After spending a short time on Tutuila, trying to pick up the Samoan language, she moved in with an American family living in a house attached to the medical dispensary on Manu'a, where she intended to carry out her fieldwork. This involved interviewing a number of young females, between 14 and 20 years of age. Based on their answers, she made a number of very specific conclusions:

(a) The Samoans were a very peaceful people.
(b) The nuclear family was of little significance. It was the extended family which held greater sway.
(c) A Samoan child had little close attachment to one person, but would cling to an aunt just as much as to its own mother.
(d) There were few social strictures limiting the freedom of a young Samoan until he or she settled down and got married. Sexual freedom was therefore tolerated, if not actively encouraged.
(e) There was absolutely no stress associated with the passage through adolescence. In fact, that was the most carefree period of a young Samoan's life.
(f) As a result of this upbringing, a young Samoan exhibited none of the anti-social behaviour which was so typical of adolescents in all western societies.

Bundling all these factors together, Margaret Mead concluded that they demonstrated a clear 'negative instance', proving that disruptive behaviour in the young was not genetically programmed, but was clearly a result of culture and environment.

Her book 'Coming of Age in Samoa' was published to great acclaim and was accepted with virtually no challenge. It became *the* anthropological textbook for the next half a century and is still considered as such in many American universities.

Already, after my short time on Tokelau, I could see how she had been misled. She had been a young American and rather naïve. She had chosen not to live with the Samoans and so did not understand them. She had arrived in a society and in an environment which she failed to comprehend. In particular she did not realise that the Samoan people were always anxious to please and this meant telling a visitor whatever they thought the visitor wished to hear. They were so nice; they wouldn't upset a *papalagi*, and certainly not a female *papalagi*. The outcome was that there was hardly a word of truth in the information she collected. Obviously there were some who were amused to mislead her on purpose. They would have a good laugh back in their home villages. And some of them were still alive, and still laughing, at the time we visited Samoa.

Of course, at the time of her writing, all the facts were imbued with deep anthropological significance. The question of whether the young Soviet Union was correct in believing that if you altered man's environment then Man himself would alter was the subject of searing debate at the time. And this question was to be resolved by looking at some primitive peoples, such as the Samoans, who represented 'the noble savage'. Therefore the learned professors took this innocent and ingenuous girl, with no special knowledge of the South Pacific, its peoples or its language, and popped her into the middle of an American family in Samoa. They let her get on with proving what their intellects informed them must happen. Otherwise what was the purpose of the Revolution?

Imagine our surprise, when, some months later, when we were again in Samoa, we were asked our opinion of a video which had been brought in from Australia. It was called, 'Margaret Mead and Samoa. The Making and Unmaking of an Anthropological Myth', by an Australian Professor of Anthropology, Dr. Derek Freeman. He had spent several years on Samoa and had studied the people and their history for a much longer period. With specific and detailed examples, he was able to refute each of Margaret Mead's assertions. As I now saw it, he was absolutely correct.

Meanwhile, we were still awaiting the arrival of a consignment of books, which had been promised by Dr. Bolinson. He was the World Health Organisation representative for the South Pacific area. We had asked for the books before we had left Apia. "No problem," he had said, when we met him in his palatial office suite, fitted out with beautiful furniture and equipped with all modern electronic office aids: printers, copiers, computers, fax machines; and the doctor ready to fly off to a conference anywhere at a moment's notice. His promise never materialised, so he obviously could not find the time to get hold of a few lousy books for my nurses!

The following day was another holiday – for the men to play cricket. On the day after that it was the women's turn. It was to be a 'workshop day'. And what was on the agenda was a modern day morality play with the doctor (yours truly) giving a talk about Aids. This was a serious subject, but in the arena of a South Pacific atoll, it was rather a hoot. This scourge of Africa, and much of the civilised world, had not reached Tokelau and most of the people did not know what it was. There was not much enthusiasm. Even though they were told that they had to attend, their attendance could not be guaranteed, at least not without a bribe. That bribe was a film, which would be shown on the screen in the Meeting House <u>after</u> the Aids talk. Even that may not have been enough to persuade them, as there was yet another distraction. After the previous day's cricket, three of the menfolk had spent a rather boozy evening, sitting on the coral beside the lagoon and drinking themselves silly. Two of them had eventually staggered off to their homes, leaving the third one singing to himself, alone with his bottle and with the stars. The following day he was nowhere to be found. A search party was organised, but with no great urgency. After all, he could not really have gone very far.

With all this excitement I was pleasantly surprised at the size of the turn-out for the lecture. I quickly quietened them down and we got started. This itself was not completely straightforward, for everything had to be translated into Tokelauan, a Polynesian language closely related to Samoan. It was pretty heavy going. The previous day I had given a script to my translator and asked her to do the best she could. She was a worldly-wise young lady who had been educated in New Zealand. She turned out to be a pretty good interpreter. It was obvious from the audience's faces that they were getting the general idea, and, from the questions at the end, it seemed that they really had understood. Although they had initially been unhappy with my choice of interpreter, they actually thanked her, and this was praise indeed. Thanking a woman, what a day!

We had been introduced to a Mr. Balani, who had been appointed as secretary to the three *Faipule*. What on earth was the significance of that? There was also a gentleman named Mr. Bileti, who obviously did not speak a great deal of English (if any). He was introduced as T.P.S. Commissioner. We had no idea of what T.P.S. was, until it was explained to us that it referred to the Tokelauan Public Services. Both gentlemen spoke enthusiastically of all that was to be done and how it was going to be done. As usual, we decided to wait and see, although, by that time, it was more in hope than expectation.

It had been a weird sort of a day all round; even the sea was acting up, and when I went back to the house, it was lapping at the doorstep. The lagoon was very full. Nearly all the boats had been pulled right up the beach, though this hardly gives the real image. After all, the islands were only about four feet above the high tide mark, so the islands were almost entirely comprised of beaches. Looking out to the far side of the reef, the sea was a brilliant vermilion, reflecting the sun, setting in the western sky; then there was a white line where the deep ocean hit the reef.

The breakers came pounding over the reef into the lagoon and across the sand bar. The deep green of the water in the lagoon gradually became lighter as the water swept towards the shore, where the emerald hue of the water blended with the underlying brightness of the sand. The children were revelling in it. By 9 o'clock in the evening, the water was up to the top of the doorstep and there it stayed until the tide subsided.

It was shortly after this that we heard the desperately sad news of a death on Atafu, another of the atolls making up Tokelau. Any death is sad, but, according to the radio reports, this one was particularly distressing, for it concerned Dr. Tyo. She was a Nigerian doctor who had been trained in Moscow, and had been sent out to Tokelau, leaving a husband and four children back at home.

Everything had gone wrong for her. Everything had gone wrong from the beginning. She had thought that she was being sent to Tokelau to set up birth control clinics. However, when she arrived on the atoll, she had discovered that she was expected to cope with all types of medical work and surgical emergencies. She had not been trained for that kind of work. She was, in fact, expected to do the same on Atafu as I was doing on Fakaofo. However, whilst I was a volunteer, who could, if so inclined, leave at any time, she was a paid employee, bound by a contract. To make it worse, she was virtually isolated from the people. Whilst I had the invaluable support of my wife, Dr. Tyo was alone and isolated in her living quarters and the hospital. She desperately wanted to get off the atoll and get back to Apia. She had last been heard on the radio, begging Dr. Liutta, the Medical Director, to take her off the atoll, a request which he had apparently refused. It seemed that, in a state of deep depression, she had killed herself. If, as seemed likely, this was all true, then I was the only medically qualified person on the three atolls, the only doctor within 400 kilometres of anywhere.

Later the ship's captain, John, came in with his wife Neta. Yes, it was all true concerning Dr. Tyo. John had just had a crazy conversation with our Medical Director, who had instructed him to take his boat up to Atafu, immerse Dr. Tyo's body in a bath of formaldehyde, and take it back to Western Samoa. I had to tell him that I could not help him out with the formaldehyde, nor did I think that he would find any on Tokelau – nor did I think that there was sufficient alcohol to pickle her in. "That's what I told Dr. Liutta," said John, "but he would not listen." In the end, John borrowed the largest freezer he could find, stuffed Dr. Tyo's body into it, loaded it onto the Tutolu and set sail from Atafu to Samoa. Apparently all this activity had been initiated by the W.H.O., who were demanding the body for a post-post-mortem.

We could not understand this, until we realised that there were probably political ramifications to the demise of the doctor. Half the Pacific seemed to have heard her pleading to be allowed to leave the atoll, and had heard Dr. Liutta refusing to listen to her pleas. He had also refused her request to speak to Dr. Bolinson, who, as head of the W.H.O. for the South Pacific area, had the ultimate responsibility. Someone was going to have to do some fancy dancing.

As Dr. Sakeya on Nukunonu was still on extended sick leave (gone to be dried out), I now really was the only qualified doctor on any of the three atolls.

From Doctor to Pathologist

That night, just after going to bed and still mulling over the implications of what had occurred, we were surprised by a loud knocking at the door. "Come quickly, doctor. The boat is waiting." I pulled on some clothes and hurried outside. There I recognised Nurse Leki, heading for the quay, which was virtually outside our front door. She was carrying a pile of white sheets from the hospital and I immediately had a premonition of what this must mean. It had to be the islander who had disappeared a couple of days earlier. It was clear that he had been found – and I was needed to examine the body, and to make certain that there had been no foul play. I climbed into the boat and we set off. The body was on the other side of the lagoon lying in a shallow pool in the coral. I did as thorough an examination as I could, but he had, after all, been in the water for two days. The fishes and crabs had clearly been at him, and the sea and coral had finished what the marine life had started. Still, I had to do my best to ensure that justice was done and I first removed his wristwatch to pass on to his wife. None other of his personal belongings had survived. An examination of the remains did not reveal any knife wounds. His front teeth were broken, but I decided that this was probably due to him bouncing up and down on the coral. And anyway, even in the unlikely event that he had been murdered, there would be no forensic evidence to help establish the identity of the culprit. It was more important to deal with the practical realities, such as the funeral. In this respect we were fortunate, for the body had washed up only yards away from a small island used by the Congregationalists as a cemetery, and he happened to have belonged to that church. Word had spread rapidly around the atoll and, by the time I finished my examination, nearly every adult male was present. They soon set about preparing a grave, a considerable excavation. He had been a large individual even before any bloating had taken place. At the same time we could hear the carpenter at work with his saw, constructing a coffin. Nurse Leki soon had the body respectfully draped in the hospital sheets and the women were allowed to approach. I guessed it was time for me to say a few well-chosen words to the relatives and onlookers, and take my leave. It was going to be a long night. A boat drove me back home. But there was no welcoming hot cup of tea; there was no power at that time of the night.

Bolt from the Blue

One evening, as we sat at home, enjoying our modest supper, a letter was delivered to us. It was from 'Eeoh' – the Executive Officer. We read it in amazement.
    The gist of the letter was as follows:
    "Dear Dr. Heller,
    I have with me two letters from you with very different hand writtings *(sic)* and signatures. One letter addressed to Gimaima *(his wife)* and the other addressed to Dr. Liutta. From the contents of these letters I can see that two different people wrote these letters. *(Quite possible. Sue had done all my secretarial work when I had worked as a G.P. and, as the illegibility of G.P.s' handwriting is legendary, it is probable that I would have asked her to write out the letter to Dr. Liutta.)* I am surprised to see that there is some untruth contained in the letter to Dr. Liutta,

because it is mentioned that the same letter was being sent to Gimaima, but that was not so. *(I had intimated in the letter to Dr. Liutta, that the same information – concerning the suspension – was being sent to Gimaima – and that was, in fact the content of the letter to her.)*

You mentioned to Dr. Liutta that the staff concerned 'really lack medical knowledge, incorrect giving out drugs and not willing to seek medical advice from us'. Who is this us refer to? If you are referring to you and your wife, I would like to know and find out your wife's position in the Tokelau Health Department or in the Tokelau Public Service. If Dr. Liutta has failed to inform me about your wife, I will find out from him. *(Sue had no official position on Tokelau, but this all comes down to the interpretation of Dr. Liutta's directive to me that I had complete authority over the running of the hospital on Fakaofo.)* I would like to find out more about your report that Gimaima really lack medical knowledge and that she has been giving out incorrect drugs. Please list all the drugs that were wrongly dispensed by the staff and also your proof of the lack of medical knowledge. I want this by tommorow *(sic)* so that I can make my report to the Director. *(After six weeks of observing Gimaima's performance and nursing skills, and of having requested details of her nursing qualifications without success, I was, and remain, convinced that she had no clinical skills. As regards the medication, I had received feedback as to the pills which were being distributed (without documentation) to the patients on the island of Fale.)*

Before I go on any further, I would like to inform you that….., before you contact Dr. Liutta, you consult the administration officer or the executive officer first. This is the system here in Tokelau. Please be advice *(sic)* that there are systems put down for doing things and you gust *(sic)* cant change any of these system without consulting us. *(I took this as downright insolence. I had been appointed by the Medical Director to work for, and report to, him and not for petty officials on Fakaofo.)*

…I am now wondering whether you and your wife were working in England like what your doing in Tokelau because being a proffessional *(sic)* person I have never seen such working condition like what you are doing, in Fiji or Apia. If I am correct you are working in Tokelau like a Foreman and a leading hand. You are the foreman and your wife the leading hand, over-ruling the senior staff nurse and the nurses. Don't ever compare Tokelau with Africa because what is happening in Africa is evil. Colonialism is evil and has long left our shores. *(His reference to Africa convinced us that he must have been accessing all our mail, as it was only in letters to Steve that we had referred to our earlier visit to Africa, although not in any way as a comparison with colonialism.)*

…Yesterday I came across your letter to Dr. Liutta, informing him about your new community worker, despite the fact that the Faipule disallowed this. I have instructed my staffs to hold on to this until the Salamasina arrived and to send by mail with my version from the council's ruling. *(I was incensed at the blatant acknowledgement that he was intercepting my mail, but, as to the appointment of the community worker, I had had nothing to do with that. It was the decision of Dr. Liutta back in Apia.)*

Coming back to Gimaima's suspension, please note that no one can suspend any public servants without prior approval from his or her superior, who are the directors. *(This was 'making policy on the hoof'. It was true for sackings, but not to my knowledge for suspensions.)*

I am sorry for the incident but there are questions to ask and reasons to hear. Gimaima has told me that these antagonistic and intransigent attitudes were towards your wife only, because you failed to explain her position in relation to the staffs of the hospital. As to the dereliction of duty, she (Gimaima) states that she work 24hrs a day seven days a week, as she is still called to dispense drugs and medicines as her nurse aid is not allowed to do so. *(This is simply a failure by the E.O. or Gimaima to face the truth: she was lazy and unreliable and would certainly not respond to a call to dispense medicines 'out of hours'. It also carefully avoids the central issue of feigning sickness so as to carry out her own private business when she should have been on duty at the hospital.)*

I am only too happy to discuss with you <u>alone</u> anything you wish to know or any help you need. I remind you again that your wife cannot sign for store supplies. If you cannot sign, ask the senior staff nurse and not your wife again.

Yours sincerely
Malima
(Executive Officer)

It was clear that he had been intercepting our private correspondence – our communications with Samoa, our letters to Steve and our correspondence with the Medical Director, and now he was demanding that we go and explain ourselves to him. We were astounded. It is hard to describe our feelings. We felt like getting away immediately. Perhaps we could take the next boat out. In a situation where the doctor on one atoll had committed suicide, where a second had left the island for treatment for alcoholism, and where we were the only qualified medical staff left, it was inconceivable that he should send such a letter. He had done his best, since we had arrived, to obstruct our work, to insult us and to block any improvements we had tried to introduce, but that was nothing compared with this latest intervention. We were in a furious mood when we eventually retired for the night. We would definitely be going on leave in February and we doubted that we would be coming back.

By the following morning, we had cooled down a little, but were still very upset. I decided to go and speak to Melli, our *Faipule*. He was incensed by the implications of my communications being revealed to anyone else, but, on the other hand, he was not really surprised, as letters were always transmitted by radio. He, himself, always waited until there was no one left in the building before establishing radio contact. After our experience, I could now understand why. We had obviously been too trusting, never dreaming that the radio operators might have been passing our transmissions to the E.O.

Soon after I had returned home, we had a visit from Melli's daughter. She had ostensibly come over for some medical advice, but really it was to exchange gossip. We showed her the letter from the E.O., which had caused us such anguish. She was horrified at its contents. Her problem was that she had been educated in N.Z. and had just been asked if she would come back to Tokelau to work. Nothing was definite, but then, as we had learnt to our sorrow, nothing was ever definite on Tokelau. She had been promised a computer by the next year, but even she had her doubts about this.

Later on Dr. Zona called in. We had a long discussion about nothing in particular, but we determined that we would go fishing, swimming and holiday-making on the following Tuesday.

There was to be a meeting of the Elders the following morning to discuss the letter that we had received from the E.O. and which had caused us such anguish. We had, of course, shown it to the *Faipule*, but not to any one else. Dr. Zona had not seen the letter, but knew of it. I explained to him that I would accept an apology in private. Face is everything, and I had no wish for the E.O. to lose face in front of the whole village. But I would also require a letter of resignation from his wife. I had had enough of her trouble making. As I saw it, they needed us and we did not really need them. And so there the matter rested, for the moment… as also did we, until about 9 o'clock in the evening.

It was at that time that another pregnant lady was brought to the hospital. We had come to accept that most expectant mothers would only come to the hospital, if they thought it really necessary and that was the case on this occasion. After all, the lady knew the ropes. She was a 'para five', having had five previous deliveries. Despite her anxieties, there were no complications and within 15 minutes she had more or less delivered herself. After that I gave her an injection to help her expel the afterbirth or placenta and she lay there on the delivery bed happily massaging her tummy to help the process. The baby didn't really interest her; it was, after all, just another girl. She refused my offer to stitch her up, on the grounds that that would give her man too much pleasure. He had had enough pleasure of her already. During our stay on Tokelau we had been surprised at how few signs of open affection were shown between the married couples. During this delivery, my wife, Sue, had acted as my assistant. In fact, I think that she probably did more work than I did, there being no other helper in the hospital at that time of night. The mother was delighted with the Papalagi woman and immediately named the baby Mini Sue.

Sue insisted I got weighed this morning, interesting, I have gone down from twelve stone and seven pounds to eleven stone and seven pounds, a loss of 14 pounds; no wonder I am feeling so good.

It was 18th January and Sue was counting the days until we could leave. The only problem was, we did not know when that would be. There was a sort of schedule for the boat, but it was notoriously unreliable.

There was another flash storm in the afternoon, which meant a frantic dashing around to close all the louvres, even though we still had the storm curtains up. We had got fed up with having to dash out in the middle of the night to drop them. If they were not dropped quickly enough, and if the wind were in the wrong direction, then the rain came roaring through the closed slats straight into our bedroom. We didn't mind the shower; our objection was to the wet bed.

By 9 o'clock in the morning everything was hot and dry again, or as dry as it was going to get. With the constant high humidity, everything always seemed damp. Sue had to keep an eye on the clothes in the wardrobe; if she left the doors closed, mould would start to grow on them. On one occasion she tried drying the washed sheets in front of the hot oven with the door open, but they soon began to smell of cooked cloth, so the idea was abandoned.

It wasn't only the problem of the damp, Sue also had to make sure that the suitcases containing our other clothes were kept closed, after she found that cockroaches liked to crawl inside and hide in the clothing.

The Elders had been meeting all day, and there were fresh rumours every time a boat came across the lagoon. The latest story was that the W.H.O. (the World Health Organisation), were going to send investigators to Atafu to try and find out what had been going on over there. We would have loved to be able to talk to them, but I had no doubt that they would be kept well away from us.

The next day there was another meeting of the Elders, but this time we were invited to attend. When we arrived at the Meeting House, the meeting had already started. It must have been the first time they had ever started anything on time; it was very odd. Melli was well into his stride, giving a résumé of why the meeting had been called, which was basically to discuss my situation. Then two other Elders reiterated the *Faipule's* words and invoked the Almighty's blessings on the meeting. They asked me to forgive them if they had misunderstood anything I had tried to do for them. 'They were, after all, just children, and we must forgive little children'. My temper was beginning to rise at all this claptrap and hypocrisy. Eventually I was given the nod to address the meeting. By now I well understood the procedure in these gatherings. First of all I thanked them for allowing me to be present at their meeting and agreed that this was only because our wise and Almighty God had decreed it so. He had guided them in their thoughts. I then went on to remind them that, where Sue and I came from, we read the same book, and that our people had been the first to bring them The Book; that the Lord's Prayer started with the words 'Our Father'; not My Father, or Your Father; but '**Our Father'**; and so on and so on for the appropriate length of time; and then into the real stuff. I explained the importance of my wife to my work. Sue and I worked as a team, together. "Whom God hath joined together let no man try to separate." I described how she had been an administrator for doctors for many years, and knew their needs and methods. I rolled off my name and my medical qualifications, and slapped onto the table copies of my qualifications. I then put down my letter of authorisation from the Apia office. After that, in a rather hurt voice, I said, "This is the second time I have been asked who I am, and by what right have I come to Tokelau. On Christmas Eve there was a meeting at the hospital. The whole staff, together with your *Pulenu'u* and your *Faipule*, attended it. These same questions were asked then, by the same two people who are asking them now; or, at least, they are now being asked by the husband of one of them. 'No, Mr. Executive Officer, there is no point in you shaking your head.' On Christmas Eve I understood that all these questions had been asked and answered. But what about the questions which I asked and to which I received no answers, and have still received no answers? By what right do these two women call themselves Staff Nurses? I am still waiting, even now, to be shown proof of their qualifications, just as I have shown you proof of mine, not once, but twice. And I am still waiting to be shown proof that they even have first aid certificates! I am tired of listening to the complaints of the patients concerning the actions and attitudes of these two people. I do not wish to be ungracious and will give praise where praise is due. Over Christmas, when we were very short staffed, we all had to work very hard. Tocina, too, worked hard and was offered a week's leave to rest and recuperate. After that, it was back to work. I recommenced my afternoon lectures, but, just as before, Tocina and Gimaima would interrupt my lectures by asking who I was; what knowledge I had; and what was I doing there. One morning Gimaima, who is married to your Executive Officer, claimed to have the 'flu. As she said she was too ill to work, I allowed her to go home. Later that day I found her cleaning out a guesthouse. She was too sick to work in the hospital but not too sick to scrub floors. She could have tried cleaning the hospital, or her filthy clinic rooms. I felt that I had no option but to suspend her from nursing duties. If I had had my way, I would have sacked her there and then." "You could not sack her" interjected the E.O. "No one can be sacked without the agreement of the New Zealand administrator. That's the law!" I pointed out that I had not sacked anyone. I had suspended the Staff Nurse from duty and that was all.

But that was not all. I then went on to relate a long list of her other inadequacies and of complaints from patients. Finally I came to the matter of the letter. "I have received a letter, a letter written by your Executive Officer, a letter so insulting to my wife and myself, that I felt that we had to let you, the Elders, know of its contents." The E.O. was now shaking his head furiously, and this was where I showed my naivety. I allowed him to interrupt me. "There is no need to show them the letter," he said. "I have given them a copy." And I, like a child, believed him and left the meeting, leaving the Elders to decide whether what I had done was right or wrong. What I did not know was that the E.O. had rewritten his letter, and it was this altered version which he had given to the Elders. Of course, the Elders could not understand what all the fuss was about, and, for our part, Sue and I were equally bemused as to why there appeared to be so little reaction from the Elders. I felt I had explained the situation quite well and the letter would have demonstrated very clearly how I had been abused.

It was days later, when we found out about the duplicity of the E.O. and of his alteration of the letter. It was Neta, captain John's wife, who gave us the news. Her father was one of the Elders and he had asked her to pass on a message. She explained that the E.O. had, on the pretext of translating the letter into Tokelauan, totally altered the context, before presenting it to the meeting. He had read it to the Elders after we had left. This accounted for the absence of any reaction by the Elders after the meeting. They had been totally misled. The truth can only have come to light through the intervention of the *Faipule*. He was the only one to have seen both the original letter and the 'translation'.

I realised that it was now too late to reconvene the meeting of the Elders. In any case, I could not recall the Elders; it had not been my meeting; they had invited me to speak to them. I had blown it!

Later this evening, in very low spirits, I went over to speak with Zona, to tell him that it was over. We had decided to go out on the next boat. We would take our holiday, as planned, and then see if there was any work in Samoa. It was a bad night for both of us. I should have asked to see the so-called letter.

Making the Best of Things

We had made up our minds, but life had to go on. It would be weeks before the arrival of the next boat.

We trundled off to the store. It wasn't exactly a shop, more like a kiosk with a counter. You had to stand at the counter, write on a piece of paper what it was you required and hand it to the person on the other side. They would then look on the few shelves to see if they had what you wanted. Sometimes they did, but more often there was very little available, except beer and cigarettes. However, we managed to get a few things and paid with our New Zealand money. We then went off to the radio transmitter and handed in our usual pointless request for drugs from Apia. We found our boatman, and sailed back home.

There were workers busy around the hospital. Due to Sue's pestering, paint, timber, piping and guttering had miraculously arrived. The place was a hive of activity. These were obviously skilled craftsmen at work! In the operating theatre we watched a painter as he carefully painted around an old calendar and then over the top of a gecko, which had unfortunately moved more slowly than his brush. I suppose it is still there, fixed in yellow paint. The rest of the workers were similarly busy, all busy at what we would call 'bodging'.

By nine in the morning the whole atoll seemed to know that we were leaving. Those we knew would give us a word of sympathy or regret. Others would whisper to each other and look away.

A message, in the form of a radiogram, had just been delivered, informing us that money had been made available to us by a Mr. Hazell and his group, back home in Wakefield, for the purchase of a large fridge freezer. It was a generous gesture, but what was the point? We were not allowed to run the hospital generator when the island generator was switched off. Therefore anything left in the freezer would be subjected to a continuous cycle of freeze and defrost, not ideal conditions, either for drugs or for food. Later we received another message; this time from Steve. He informed us that he had acted on the message and had ordered the freezer. This was in spite of the fact that we had previously talked it over with him and explained why we did not think that it was a particularly good idea. We cabled Mr. Hazell to stop any further monies being sent until we had had a chance to review the situation. I was certain that, if we went ahead with the order, the freezer would end up in someone's house in Samoa.

It was a splendid day, apart from the deep depression in which we found ourselves. However, at last, and after many promises, Dr. Zona and wife chose that day to take us out. Not only were we to be taken on a picnic, but we would be taken on a boat trip around the whole atoll. We took with us both our still cameras and the camcorder, with all the batteries fully charged. The damned batteries were always flat. I suppose it was the temperature – or the humidity. Surely the Japanese were capable of producing a battery for use in that climate. It turned out to be a glorious day and just the thing to take our minds off our other woes. Sue ended up getting sunburnt. It was a lovely day. We stopped and landed at one very small islet where there was a small hut and a large sheltered area. This, Zona explained, was their honeymoon island, to which newly weds retired after the ceremony and the feast. Dr. Zona's daughter, Leki, had prepared a most sumptuous meal. Admittedly the sandwiches contained corned beef and tinned fish (to which I had a certain aversion, as explained earlier), but the bread was home baked, and it was beautiful. Leki had also baked a cake with a thick covering of sticky icing. I don't know how they had managed to obtain all the ingredients.

By now we had been joined by Zona's young grandchild and his friend; they had sailed over in another outboard. The water as always was beautifully warm and so we swam. After some time, Dr. Zona suggested that we sailed on and he would give us a guided tour of all the other little islands. As he explained, he had not been around the atoll himself since before the last hurricane, which had been some years earlier. It was an amazing afternoon. He pointed out the places where the islanders would come for the big crabs. Officially, one could only come for these if there was to be a special feast, as there had been when we first arrived on the atoll, but it seemed that whenever someone fancied crab for a snack, then crab would mysteriously appear on the table. There was another tiny islet, which Zona recalled as having been covered by trees. That was before the storm. Now it was completely bare. And so we passed the day, with Sue and me being fascinated by Zona's tales. It was amazing to think that on such a small atoll, people were not aware of what was happening on the other side of the lagoon. Even Zona, who was one of their best fishermen and fished every other day, was unfamiliar with some of the smaller islands. It had been a good day.

We had not been home more than 10 minutes when Neta arrived and told us that John and Steve were on the R/T. Sue went off to have a chat; it's amazing how voice lonely one could get.

The next day being a Sunday, the power came on early for church. We had carefully avoided going to any church services, so as to avoid any perception that we might favour either one of the two main religious groups, the Congregationalists and the Roman Catholics. Since arriving on the atoll, we had been somewhat perplexed to find that the leader of the Catholics had a wife and eight children. This went against everything we knew about the Catholic clergy. However, we had finally figured out that he was not actually a priest. He was what they called a catechist. We had already learned that they had no proper doctors (except for myself) and no proper nurses, but now it seemed that they had no proper ministers either.

I went outside, from where I could see the school boat heading for the jetty. As the school was on our island, but the main centre of population was on the smaller island, a boat had been supplied to transport the children to and from school. It therefore plied its way back and forth across the lagoon and, when not being used for the schoolchildren, would be commandeered by others, particularly important visitors. That is how I came to observe Mr. Balani, the recently installed secretary to the three *Faipule*, waving to me as he trotted off the boat at the jetty. He wanted to know if he could come over that evening for a chat. It was odd; still, I said he should come round at about eight. In the meantime, I went over to have a chat to Zona, to thank him for such a wonderful excursion, but also to tell him that we had not changed our minds. We still intended to leave on the next boat, whenever that should be. We had had enough. We came here to run a hospital, not to get mixed up in a load of bickering and island politics. We had decided that we would go back to Samoa, have a holiday, and then see if there was any chance of picking up any work over there. It would be great to have a holiday, a real holiday; to go somewhere that we could flick a switch so that the light would come on; to have clean water straight from the tap; and no big insects to think about. Having made up our minds to leave, we had all the time in the world.

On the atoll was one family from the Gilbert Islands, very much darker in colour than the native islanders, or even the Samoans. They were considered as very much the poorer relations, though it was difficult to see how any one could be much poorer than any one else. No, that's not true, there were very fine lines of distinction, based on the backgrounds of the different families. Gred, our Gecko painter, was considered to be among the upper stratum. He was very well connected. He was also very idle. He loved to sit in his *fale*; to order the females around, whilst they ministered to his every whim. He had gout, though that did not stop him drinking. He demanded tablets for the pain, so that he could continue drinking and at the same time he sent his wife to the hospital to obtain a sick note proving that he was unfit to work. There are, unfortunately, people like that in every society.

The main work was the repair of the lagoon walls. It was strange to see them building up and repairing the walls on the lagoon side of our islands and not on the ocean side. It was the ocean side which took the heaviest battering during a storm.

As arranged, Mr. Balani arrived to have a talk. We had no idea what the subject of the discussion would be, although it was common knowledge on the atoll that a discussion with Mr. Balani usually meant listening to and agreeing with everything he had to say. It turned out to be another very frustrating meeting, which reminded me rather of Alice in Wonderland:

"I quite agree with you," said the Duchess; "and the moral of that is – 'Be what you would

seem to be' – or, if you'd like it put more simply – 'Never imagine yourself not to be otherwise than what it might appear to others that what you were or might have been was not otherwise than what you had been would have appeared to them to be otherwise.'" "I think I should understand that better," Alice said very politely, *"if I had it written down."*

We could make about as much sense of the peroration of Mr. Balani. However, rather than us asking him to write it down, as Alice had done, we were amazed when he ended by asking whether I had written everything down, by which he meant everything which had been said at the meeting in the Meeting House the previous day. I expressed my surprise that he, as Secretary to the *Faipule*, had not made a record of the meeting. And even if he had not done so, then surely the Executive Officer would have made a note of everything. Oh, no; that appeared not to be the case, and he wanted yet another list of the failings of the medical staff. I emphasised that he had in his possession a letter in which I had explained why I had felt it necessary to suspend the two nurses, and I did not feel it necessary to keep on repeating myself. He was not satisfied with that. He wanted it in my own handwriting. By this time I was beginning to lose my patience. What on earth was behind it all? As patiently as I could, I explained that if he wished to be able to read what was written, then he had better accept a report written in my wife's handwriting, which I would then sign. Her writing was at least legible. At that point we ended the meeting. It was time for us to make our nightly rounds of the patients. I'm sure that he would never have thought of that. Patient care was the last thing in his mind.

Earlier in the day, before my attention had been distracted by the arrival of Mr. Balani, I had received a visit from the *Faipule*'s wife. She brought us a gift of a fish large enough to feed us for at least a week. However, it soon became clear that the main purpose of her visit was to consult me on a professional basis. She explained that, while she had been in New Zealand, she had been treated for tuberculosis. Unfortunately, although she was supposed to stay on the medication for at least a year, they had not given her enough tablets. She would have come to see me earlier, she said, but she had waited to see if she could trust me. She had finally decided that she could. To what extent that decision had been prompted by my actions, rather than by the fact that she had now run out of drugs, was never clear to me. What I did find surprising was that this was the wife of Melli, the *Faipule*, whom I had always considered to one of the more supportive members of the community. The fact that she had not been prepared to trust me showed just how insular the population was. I was trying to think what I could prescribe for her, when I recalled that, a couple of weeks before, Sue had, during one of her 'Operation Clear-out' sessions on the hospital cupboards, discovered a large supply of drugs for the treatment of tuberculosis. As I had still not, until that day, been aware of any incidence of T.B. on the atoll, this had gone out of my mind. The predicament of the *Faipule*'s wife reminded me of the find and I was able to give her sufficient tablets to complete her course of treatment. Before leaving she stressed that everything she had said had to be kept in the Most Absolute Confidence. (If she ever reads this diary, I hope she will forgive me!)

The following day we received a visit from Staff Nurse Yanetta. She has not previously figured in this story, as she was not a close associate of those whom I considered the conspirators, namely Tocina and Gimaima. She too had probably gained Staff Nurse status due to length of service, being about 40 years old, but she had always shown enthusiasm and eagerness to learn. She realised how little they all knew about nursing. She wanted to progress to a standard where she might gain employment in New Zealand. She was ambitious not only for herself but also for her children, and hoped that eventually she might be able to afford a good education for them. Incidentally, she was still breast-feeding her youngest child, who was about 18 months old, and it was fascinating to watch her go about her ward duties carrying her baby on her hip.

Anyway, on that afternoon, Yanetta had come to see me because of the rumours, which were rife in the hospital. She wanted to hear it 'from the horse's mouth'. Were we going to leave? She was very upset, when we explained our decision to her and she returned to the hospital in tears.

I couldn't get Mr. Balani out of my mind. His visit of the previous evening was still bugging me. I had tried to explain the reasons for my actions, but I was clearly wasting my time. He had just wanted me to agree to 'forgive and forget', to forget the very reason that all this trouble had blown up. It was of no interest to him who was in the right and who in the wrong. Nor did it matter that the issues I had raised were very serious, affecting the health and well-being of the islanders themselves. As far as he was concerned, they had managed quite well before I had arrived, without being confronted with all this aggravation. Admittedly, if I had not come, a few more people may have passed away and a few less babies may have survived, but, after all, that was God's will! Warming to his theme, Mr. Balani not only asked me to forgive the two Staff Nurses, but also to give them special tuition. I managed to keep my temper under control while I explained how ludicrous it would be to waste resources on these two individuals, both of whom were near the end of their careers, while there were eager young nurses desperate to improve their skills. But in this society, youth was not a factor to be considered and Mr. Balani ignored the suggestion. He just continued his defence of the two Staff Nurses. He once again re-iterated the point that no employee could be dismissed except by order of the New Zealand authorities. I had no idea whether there was any truth in this or whether he, and all the others in apparently senior positions, made up the rules and regulations as they went along. I was not even sure of Mr. Balani's position or authority. Whenever I raised the question, I was fobbed off. I assumed that he did have some authority, but I was not sure how far it reached. Anyway, any discussion of 'dismissal' was academic, as I had not dismissed anyone, I had only suspended them.

Since the previous day's unpleasant and unsatisfactory meeting with Mr. Balani, I had learned that he was to address yet another meeting of the islanders that evening, apparently to spell out to everyone what they could and could not do. He wanted to emphasise that he was the person in authority, once and for all. I was still feeling exhausted from our meeting, so had no wish to listen to him again. In any case the meeting was to be held in the local language, so that let me off the hook.

I do know that I gave even greater attention than normal to the preparation of my tutorial session with the nurses that afternoon. I was certainly not going to give them any more ammunition to fire back at me and I was keen to emphasise the point that I was the only trained medical resource they had. Driving Sue and me from the atoll would hurt them far more than it would hurt us.

The following day we began to hear reports of Balani's meeting. He had apparently told the islanders that 'the only authority now was his'. Everything must be done with his leave. Even the Elders were deprived of their traditional authority, at least according to him. In particular, he stressed that no employee could be hired or fired without his agreement. I suspect that this bit had been added for my benefit. If so, he would have been pleased that it was reported back to me so quickly!

I spoke with Dr. Liutta later on in the day over the radio link. I kept it all very light and superficial. He asked how we were getting on with the people. I informed him quite truthfully that we had a very good relationship, not only with the *Faipule* and the *Pulenu'u*, but also with the people in general, especially our patients. Maybe I chickened out of a confrontation with him, but we had already made up our minds on our future plans and had nothing to gain from mentioning Mr. Balani and the Executive Officer. I gained the impression that he was grateful that I didn't involve anyone else, but I was equally sure that he was well aware of exactly what was going on. Very briefly we went over the plans for our forthcoming holiday, but only to the same extent as we had discussed with him previously. We would go back to Apia for a short while and then visit New Zealand. We didn't mention our decision not to return to Tokelau and he didn't ask. We felt that we had upset enough people.

On returning to my desk, I looked for some papers, on which I had been working, and discovered that they were missing. In fact, a considerable number of my papers had disappeared. Thinking back, I realised that I had last seen them before the meeting with Mr. Balani. He must have taken them with him. I could only hope that it had been unintentional. Reluctant as I was to speak to him again, I would have to confront him on the matter.

Sue was very depressed. She was finding everything very stressful. It was only the thought that we would soon be leaving, which was holding her together. She cherished the prospect of a long holiday, on our own, with no one else to please but each other. With no plans to return to Tokelau, we were free to plan a longer visit to New Zealand, rather than a quick flit around the country. We would be able to explore the wine trails, to visit friends. We might even have time to visit Julian, a fellow doctor, who had emigrated to New Zealand after living and working very close to our home in Yorkshire. It was hard to believe that all this was now within our grasp.

I had another bad night. I was restless and couldn't sleep. Suddenly I thought I heard someone padding about. In my drowsy state, my only thought was for my diary. I struggled out of bed, convinced that someone was trying to steal my writings. Was I going paranoid, or was it my nerves beginning to wear a little thin? Looking back, it was probably the knowledge that Balani had taken some of my papers away with him which was preying on my mind. My restlessness awoke Sue, who thought it must be one of our maternity patients going off home. As with all patients, she could discharge herself whenever she wished, but we did not expect her to leave in the middle of the night. I had hoped to weigh and check over her baby before she left. I had suspected that it might not be getting enough nutrition. Sure enough, when I did my ward round in the morning, her bed was empty. She had gone home.

At about eight in the morning I stopped Balani as he was walking along the beach towards the jetty, intending to board the school boat. We exchanged pleasantries and then I asked him to open his brief case. He must have seen that I was in no mood to argue and he opened the case. Immediately I saw what I was looking for and I grabbed my papers. He showed no surprise that the papers had been in his bag and made no attempt to apologise. On the contrary, he was clearly frustrated at having to return them to me. It was obvious that it had not been an oversight when he had swept all my papers together with his own notes into his folder. Any remaining trust I had in Mr. Balani was fast disappearing.

I had time later that morning to have a look at how the workers were progressing. They must have started on a second coat of paint, as the five-year-old calendar, which Gred had so carefully painted around, was now completely painted over. The gecko was still entombed! We had hoped that a number of broken electrical sockets would be renewed, or at least repaired, but no; they were also just painted over. Some new guttering was being put up and they had some new piping on site.

Within a day or two, I was feeling sufficiently recovered from the exhaustion of the previous nights to set about compiling the report requested by Mr. Balani. Had it been just for his benefit, I would probably have ignored the request, but if there was any chance of improving the hospital facilities, then I felt a moral obligation to do my best. The report covered a wide range of topics, such as:

    a) The current health of the population
    b) The current facilities available in the hospital
    c) The potential for expanding the hospital services
    d) The current staffing situation
    e) Current and future staff requirements
    f) Staff training
    g) Equipment and maintenance requirements
    h) Any problems which I anticipated.

It was a pretty tall order, but I did my best. I would have been interested to know whether he really wanted my help or was just impatient to get me off the atoll. He must have realised that without outside expertise the medical situation could only deteriorate, but did that concern him at all? I had no way of knowing.

I was still immersed in my report, when captain John arrived with some mail. He was in a hurry, as usual. He intended to pick up Neta and take her with him on a trip to the other two atolls. I envied her. I felt sorely tempted to throw down my pen, call Sue to pack a bag, and jump on the boat. But I was a doctor and simply too conscientious.

In the Doldrums

The mail turned out to consist mainly of Christmas cards. These had been posted round about 8th December. It was now approaching the end of January, so Christmas was long since forgotten. I am not one for Christmas cards and did not appreciate all the pseudo-religious nonsense. However, given a choice, I think that I preferred the most obsequious Christmas card to the seasonal greeting sent to us by the Lancashire and Yorkshire Friendly Society. The Society was the guardian of some of our savings. After all, friendly societies are 'as safe as houses', as the saying goes; except this one, of course. The Lancashire and Yorkshire had decided to invest in property, right at the peak of the boom – and just before someone had pointed out that their articles of incorporation did not allow their funds to be invested in property. By this time, inevitably, the bottom had dropped out of the property market. We were powerless. Even a letter of complaint would probably not reach them before they went bust, or had, at least been the target of a buy-out. We resigned ourselves to the fact that we would be lucky to get anything back from our investment. Perhaps we should have just put our money into a building society. It probably served us right.

It was at about 5 o'clock in the evening on the following day; our last patient had finished her washing and gone home, taking her new baby Mini Sue with her; when Yanetta came in to see me. She wished to introduce her husband. They lived on the other island, where he worked as one of the two radio operators. I thought he might wish to discuss Yanetta's health, as I had recently diagnosed her as being not only diabetic, but also as suffering from hypertension – and all this while still breast-feeding her small child. However, this was not the case, he rather wished to add his voice to the increasing concern as the news spread that we were leaving Tokelau. He had also brought us some news; Steve and Ava were now married. I wondered how they had reconciled their wish for a quiet wedding with the demands of their society for a typical Samoan celebration. We would have to wait until we saw them again for an answer to that question.

We were still digesting the news brought by Yanetta's husband, when we had a further supplication, this time from Leki's husband. Leki was the daughter of Dr. Zona and also the most competent of the nurses working in the hospital. We therefore had a lot of respect for her and her family. Nevertheless we were rather surprised that her husband would come to see us, particularly when it became clear that his was yet another plea for us to stay on Fakaofo and not to leave Tokelau. However, the request was more personal than a simple request to consider the interests of the atoll. He was anxious that his wife's pregnancy should have proper medical supervision. If we were determined to leave, then would it be possible for Leki and him to come and stay with us? He would save up to pay the fare. It was all a pipe dream. Leki's husband had never been off the atoll, let alone visited England or even Samoa. He would know a little about New Zealand, as Leki had spent some time there, and probably envisaged England as being part of the same land mass. His pay was ridiculously low, as was that of Leki, so the chance of them saving any money was minimal. I was very sympathetic and did not wish to disillusion him. After all, Leki must have recognised the reality of their situation. She had been abroad and had a wider appreciation of the world. She was in an awkward situation. Her father had been ostracised, because of his religious views, and some of the distrust was still directed at her. When there had been an opportunity of a scholarship for a nurse to take an anaesthetic course on Fiji, Leki had been ruled out by the Elders, despite being clearly the most suitable applicant. She was a trained midwife and she was intelligent. It would have all fitted in nicely. Perhaps they were right in thinking that she would not have returned to Tokelau after the course, but that risk applied to most of the islanders given the chance to travel abroad. Whatever the reason, Dr. Liutta was prevailed upon to nominate a person with no training whatsoever. All we could offer as encouragement to Leki and her husband was the suggestion that they might apply to a police training college back in the U.K. We knew that they had taken on both Samoan and Fijian police officers, so maybe that was a possibility – especially in the land of dreams.

Although I often considered Tokelau, cut off so completely from reality, as being a land of dreams, Sue did not see it in the same light. She was no longer even able to get a decent night's sleep, let alone have pleasant dreams. Every little noise would disturb her; the wind whistling around the tin roofs, the lapping of the water on the shore, or the aluminium boats banging together beside the jetty; everything would unsettle her. One continuing reason for her unease was the death of Dr. Tyo. Sue still felt very bitter about the way in which the doctor had been abandoned. This feeling was further aggravated by the verdict of the inquest that her death had been caused by an accidental overdose. Obviously this suited everyone – except someone interested in getting at the truth. The death had been an accident, so no blame could be attached to anyone. There need be no loss of face. We realised that there might be other factors, such as any insurance claims by Dr. Tyo's dependants, but it did seem to be a very convenient way out for those responsible.

Morning dawned at last, bright and clear as usual, and I went out for a stroll along the beach, taking my camera. I was particularly interested to photograph the canoe of Dr. Zona, in which we had so recently sailed around the atoll. It was one of the few remaining wooden outriggers on the atoll. The main hull was not made from an entire tree trunk, as we had seen in other parts of the South Pacific, but was built up of relatively short pieces of wood, which had been shaped and then glued and stitched together. This was a far more complicated method of construction than that using an entire tree trunk, but it seemed that the atolls of Tokelau had been depleted of the necessary type of trees many years earlier.

The people of Tokelau had become increasingly generous to us. Among many other things, we had been given two magnificent clam shells, each one about a foot across and very beautiful. We envisaged some difficulty in getting them back into England, but Sue was adamant, "They are coming back home with us and that's that!"

Our diet had also improved enormously due to the generosity of the population.

We had eggs to pickle, beautiful bread from Zona's wife and a tasty cheese from an unknown islander. We also received gifts of fish, in particular several large bonitos, over three feet long, and, on one occasion a massive hand of bananas. This we hung from one of the veranda beams, hoping that it would ripen. The people of Tokelau did not normally eat bananas as a fruit, but rather as a vegetable, which was cooked in the green state. Therefore we rarely saw a ripe yellow banana, such as we would normally buy at home.

The most recent presents had been a tin of butter and a tin of jam. Those would be very much appreciated for our afternoon tea.

I was very surprised to receive a further visit from Balani. After our last altercation I had expected that he would stay away from me. I was even more surprised when he asked me, very civilly, whether he could be taken on a tour of the hospital. This was the same Balani, who had been so keen for everyone to appreciate his power and authority. He was in charge of everything; why should he need my permission to visit the hospital? I was becoming increasingly convinced that we were living in Wonderland, even if we had still not run into Alice.

We were regular visitors to the island store. One never knew, maybe there would be something tempting in stock. What was much less usual was for the lady who ran the store to visit us. However, one afternoon she stood at our door, husband in tow. After listening to a long and convoluted story, I gathered that he was having problems with his waterworks. A short course of antibiotics would soon sort it out, except that the hospital had no antibiotics, until the arrival of the next boat. Once again I had to rely on our own private supply of drugs, which we had brought with us from England.

It was at about 6 o'clock that evening and I sat with Sue, enjoying a slice of hot buttered toast. She was fiddling with the radio, trying to pick up news from Australia. Reception was not good, but she was able to gather that there had been a serious earthquake in Los Angeles, with many people reported dead. How far away it all seemed – and how much more immediate was the hot buttered toast!

As we enjoyed our meal, Sue outlined an idea she had concerning the schoolchildren. She wanted to involve them in a campaign to improve their environment. She proposed a competition to design and paint a poster, one for each age group, with prizes for the best designs in each group. The subject of the posters was to be 'Cleaning up the Atoll'.

The next day, Sue discussed the idea with the headmaster. He was very enthusiastic and thought it a wonderful idea. The initial reaction from the children was also very promising and there was even some interest from their parents, to the extent that, over the course of the next week, an accumulation of rubbish had been collected together and piled up into a heap. It was clear that most of it was made up of rusty tin cans, many of them having previously contained tinned fish. It always made my blood boil. Here we were, sitting on a lagoon full of fish, and yet we had to import it in cans! Of course, it was not only fish, but also inferior meat and even custard. Oh, well!

At one time the atoll had exported a small amount of timber and even some fish. Now the only fish to be exported, was that taken out on the boat to relatives in Samoa or New Zealand. As for timber, there was no longer sufficient even for the modest demands of the atoll itself. The enthusiasm for the 'clean up' campaign lasted about a week – and Sue never did see any of the anticipated posters. Whether it was the children, or the headmaster, who had lost interest, she would never know. What did surprise her, was the arrival, a short time after she had suggested the project, of some cards from Samoa proposing virtually the same idea. John had brought them back with him from Apia, but had simply laid the package to one side, without even opening it.

Some good things did arrive in cans, and Sue, in particular, was very partial to a supper of tinned sago, honey and banana. I hoped it would buck her up a little.

Afterwards I read another ten pages of 'Dudley's Emergency Surgery', and then Sue questioned me about my previous readings. She nearly always went back to the same few operations, strangulated hernias, Caesarean sections and perforated ulcers. So far I had been lucky. I had had no really serious cases requiring immediate surgery. But I supposed it couldn't last forever, my luck I mean.

Mind-numbing as this home study was, it was better than the alternative – the damned radio! It just seemed to spew out continuous crappy music, not a single spoken word. This is what happened very often when Radio Samoa, for some reason or other, failed to pick up Radio Australia or New Zealand. Radio Samoa used both of these radio programmes for its own news round-ups.

That night the power stayed on until 1 o'clock in the morning. We assumed that there must be a patient being brought to the hospital from the other island, but everything remained quiet. We never discovered what had caused this change in normal practice, but the knock-on effect was that the power didn't come on again until halfway through the morning. We were left with a room full of dental patients, but no power for the drill or lights.

The following night was also disturbed, not, this time, by the generator or by the patients, but by the weather. The wind and rain were so strong that we were forced to get up and close the louvres over the windows. The morning remained grey and overcast. It was 23rd January, so should still have been summer, but this was the wet season so, relative to the usual hot clear days, it seemed like winter. At 8.30 a.m. the power was switched on and, as we sat down to toast and tea, the church bells were calling the faithful. Sue thought this a good opportunity to have a shower, before the water supply failed; the tank had not been filled for two days. What had aggravated the situation had been the fact that our last maternity case, before leaving the hospital with Mini-Sue, had completed her week's laundry. This was quite usual; it was much easier to do it at the hospital than when they arrived back at their own *fales* – and we even had washing lines strung up outside the hospital. Not only were we running very short of water, but what we had was badly contaminated. I determined that one day I would try to photograph the inside of one of the concrete water tanks.

Many islanders were now using plastic collecting tanks. It was the same dirty water running off the same dirty tin roofs, but it was nevertheless much cleaner than that which came out of our tanks. Some of the plastic tanks even had opening in the top to enable them to be cleaned out. The variety of animal life which came out of our tap was unbelievable. What a pity it was that the original fresh water supplies had been exhausted (or contaminated). Walking around the island, one still came across the rusted remains of pumps attached to the borehole pipes. We were reminded of this when, later that day, we went for a walk. We took with us some empty screw-top bottles, as we had already arranged to call in to see the family who always had a supply of fresh, beautiful-tasting water. We drank a little and exchanged a little chit-chat and then it was time for the slow stroll back home. It was really too hot for walking. For me it had been a rather embarrassing experience. I was wearing a pair of brand-new, and rather expensive, shorts. In that climate, it seemed unnecessary to wear underpants – at least, it did until I sat down, whereupon I found that my fundamentals would keep popping out. Why on earth didn't the maker, a famous manufacturer, put a jockstrap inside? I determined that I would have to go back to my grey *lava lava*, which was the attire worn by the Elders of the atolls.

On arriving home from our walk, we found that someone had dropped a hand of ripe bananas outside our door. The folk were very kind to us; they knew that Sue loved bananas. The islanders always used the diminutive for her, and already there was a growing tribe of Little Suzeys, as well as some Maxis. Sue kept a note of all their birthdays in her diary.

That evening we switched on the radio, which Zona had kindly loaned us, and were lucky to pick up a programme from Radio Australia, relayed to Tokelau by Radio Samoa. We could hardly believe that we were listening to the choir of Guildford Cathedral. They were all records, of course, but how wonderful. Sue was homesick. She was missing our home and all that went with it. It was unusual for us to be able to hear good music on the radio, and our little tape deck and tapes were nearly worn out – just as we were!

It was the following day that Sue received a big shock. On checking our airline tickets, she saw that they were incorrect. In fact, they contained not one, but two mistakes. Our intended trip to the Cook Islands had been completely omitted and there was a wrong date shown for our return flight back to the U.K. Oh well, one thing was certain; we could do nothing about it until we left Tokelau.

Meanwhile, I was still waiting for Mr. Balani to come and visit our hospital.

My suspension of Gimaima had left the clinic on the other island unmanned. I had therefore asked Yanetta to look after it. She lived over there and it seemed convenient. Subsequently I decided that it would be better to have Leki at the other clinic, so Yanetta moved back to our hospital. Leki was really the brightest of the girls, who would cope on her own. Yanetta was careful and caring, but she was still breast-feeding her youngest; and she was a diabetic with unstable blood pressure. She needed someone to guide her; but at least she was trustworthy. And at least she would say if she had not understood something. Not many of them would do that. They invariably said 'yes', and then either forgot all about it, or did what they thought you might have meant.

On another rainy and windy night, Sue had to get up (she had become the lightest of sleepers now) in order to close the louvres behind our bed. The wind had swung around and was blowing into the other window, where there was no storm curtain, so the rain just came blowing in. Above the noise of the storm, she could hear the sound of the termites; still busy eating away at the headboard. I slept on, content in the knowledge that we would be gone before they finished it. Sue had lost the spring in her step. We could only carry on and await the arrival of the boat.

When we got up the next morning, we found that someone had again left us some ripe bananas. Where on earth were they getting them from? As the islanders usually used them while they were still green, we never saw any yellow bananas on the trees. It was a real treat. There were two plastic bottles left with the bananas, one, by its taste, contained three-day old coconut juice and the other was *cava*. This was a local hallucinogenic and intoxicant. I thought that they must be trying to tell us something!

Zona came in early to have a chat and to bring some fresh pawpaws for Sue. He, and everyone, was being so nice to us. He came, he said, because he had a worry. Fakaofo was expecting a visit from Form 5 students from Nukunonu Atoll, which was the closer of the other two atolls making up Tokelau. They were to take part in a choir competition on our atoll. On Nukunonu they had a bad drug problem. They were not alone in this regard. It was a problem throughout Samoa and the South Pacific, although fortunately not yet on Fakaofo. Zona was concerned that the young people from Nukunonu might bring the habit with them. There was so little work and no prospects of improvement. Coupled with this, the introduction of video cassette players, even on those islands which had no television, meant that the islanders now had a much clearer perception of life in the rest of the world. They had no way of knowing that most of the films gave a very distorted view of what life was really like. It was inevitable that expectations would be raised, and equally inevitable that hopes would be dashed. This probably accounted for the high rate of suicide among the young people of the region.

There really was no work on Fakaofo, except the digging up of our island and the transferring of the materials to the other inhabited island. The purpose of this was to reinforce the sea wall. This, and any other work, was shared out on a rotational basis by the Public Works Department, and hence any available funds were distributed by the P.W.D.

The fact that the P.W.D. shared out the work did not mean that it would necessarily get done, as I realised as soon as Dr. Zona had departed. It was very quiet around the hospital. No workers had turned up. It was almost as if they had exhausted themselves with slapping the paint on. I took the hint and also went off for a midday siesta. I woke up just in time to give the nursing staff my afternoon lecture. Dr. Zona was also there. The subject, by popular demand, was 'Intravenous therapy – why? when? and how?'. It's amazing how much one can remember, when put to the test; the difficulty was in putting it into a language that the islanders could understand. Also I had to be careful to restrict my references to the equipment that we had in the hospital and to the fluids and medicines which we had available. There was said to be a blood register somewhere on the atoll, but no one seemed to know where it was, nor did they know their individual blood groups. In my talk I tried to encourage the staff to make decisions for themselves, especially as to who should be given the treatment, when there was only a limited amount of treatment available.

There had been a beautiful breeze all day, so Sue and I took a walk around our island, this time in a clockwise direction. We tended not to meet so many people going that way. Sue was feeling much better and wished that we could come back again, but she recognised that this would not be possible. If we were ever to return, it would be to Fakaofo. We had become attached to the atoll and its people, and we had no wish to go off to the other atolls in spite of their blandishments. It had taken us too many arguments over the R.T. to get what we had managed to obtain for the people of Faka.

When we went back inside the house, Sue switched on the radio. What did we hear? Mona Lisa; God, how old was that tune? It had been a slow day! Still, our walk had given us a healthy appetite, and we ate too much; cooked breadfruit with some cheese melted over it, some of our spiced fish and a little of our fried Bonito. It was wonderful to feel full, but it was too much for our shrunken stomachs, we found it very difficult to go to sleep. Served us right!

A Ceremonial Occasion

The next day was 28th January and Dr. Zona had indicated that he wished to come over early in the morning 'for a little chat'. It seemed that he was using me as a sounding board, enabling him to get his thoughts in order and I knew that he would be involved in meetings on both that and the following day. There was much discussion on the apparent power shift being driven by Balani and his fellow officials from New Zealand. I suspected it would be a case of 'all change, no change'.

The three *Faipule*, one from each atoll, had been delegated to set up an executive branch of the new government, the rumour was that the Council of the Elders had been assured that they would still have the final say on almost everything. I just could not believe that. Balani's manner did not suggest that he had been sent to Tokelau to play second fiddle to the Elders.

When Dr. Zona arrived, he announced that Sue and I had been invited to the Big Meeting the following day. This was clearly to be a special occasion, as indicated by the fact that it was suggested that I wear a jacket and tie. It was an honour for outsiders to be invited to such a meeting and we were aware that it would be a 'once in a lifetime' occasion. We already knew that we were the first English people to live and work on the atoll since the missionaries had visited in 1850. We did not wish to dwell on the fact that *they* had been eaten…..

For the rest of that day, we just sat around in nervous anticipation. We had little choice. That was the worst thing with my job, when there was a lull in the workload, there was little else to do. As so often, I pondered on the medical services available and what was really needed. There was no doubt that I was performing an important service, but it was no more than a very good nurse from a casualty department would have been able to handle without difficulty. The problem was that there was no such adequately trained nurse. In the hospital's jam-packed drawers, there was everything from brace and bit to skull crackers and rib spreaders, but no staff qualified to use them. This was perhaps just as well, as most of the equipment was well rusted. In fact, I think that I would have needed my skull looking into if I had considered using some of the instruments provided. I even had to use a pair of pliers to operate the valve of an oxygen cylinder, as the proper key, if there ever had been one, had disappeared. It had probably been used for some other purpose; not necessarily lost or stolen, just gone walkabout.

The burning heat had gone out of the sun; but it was still hot, too hot for Sue's comfort. I took myself off to a little place I had found, where, with the aid of a couple of large stones and my snorkel, I could sit undisturbed under the water and just watch that other world. I just wished that we had been better equipped.

At last the big day dawned. We had learned that our *Faipule* was to be made Chief of all three atolls. There was to be an all day ceremony, starting at 9.00 a.m. and going on until midnight. John's boat, the Tutolu, had been busy ferrying the *Faipule* and Elders from the other two atolls. There would be much singing and feasting. Unfortunately the ceremony would be conducted in Tokelauan, so we would understand very little of it. Nevertheless, we knew that, although it would be a long day, it would be very interesting.

We were taken in the hospital boat across the lagoon to the main island and made our way to the Meeting House. We had decided to try to video what we could of the ceremonies. However, remembering the troubles that we had previously had with our camera batteries, we could only hope. We had made sure that they were all fully charged and we were determined to have a pictorial record of the experience. The temperature was already high, and it was going up.

We entered the Meeting House at about 8.30 a.m. and each was presented with a string of shells to put around our necks, and also with a garland of flower heads. The women must have been up all night making so many garlands. We were delighted to find that, along with the *Faipule* and their wives, a few of the top Elders and ourselves were given white plastic chairs to sit on. We didn't fancy the idea of sitting cross-legged all day on the coconut mats, which now covered the entire floor.

By 2 o'clock in the afternoon, the three *Faipule*, together with nominated Elders from the three atolls, had each made speeches, as had the *pulenu'u* and a representative from New Zealand. Then, after our *Faipule* had said a few more words, he was presented with a traditional skirt of office, made from coconut leaves. We were enjoying it immensely. It was just a pity that we could not understand a word.

After that came the singing and dancing. The children from our senior school sang. Then the boys and young men danced and sang, followed by the girls. They had been practising for months. The older men followed with similar dances and singing, and lastly the women. Like many of the Pacific Islands the hand movements were elegant and distinctive. We just wished that we had had someone to interpret the dances for us. The whole celebration was clearly a very important occasion for our atoll. I hoped that Sue had managed to get some of it on video; it was such an incredible experience.

After the speeches came the food, all prepared by the ladies of the atoll. Two roast pigs were held high and paraded around the outside of the Meeting House where the ceremony was being held. The women walking on each side of the pigs were singing and waving their leaves and fans to keep the flies and insects off. The pigs were then put on trestle tables and were cut up with a very large knife. The dishes of meat were then surrounded with all the other food. The chiefs and their wives were served first, collecting their food on plates made of woven banana leaves. We followed, leading the Elders, as the Doctor was of a higher rank. Once again the food took the same format as before: green bananas cooked in coconut milk, taro, a chunk of pork, with a lot of fat, noodles in a brown sauce, a door stop of bread, and a slice of something made out of semolina, along with a number of things we couldn't identify. Coke, lemonade, and a little beer were also available. At about 6 p.m. the party broke up for an hour's rest. We decided not to bother returning to our island, so sat talking to some of the people whom we knew well. Later in the evening the dancing and singing started again and carried on until midnight. The atmosphere was electrifying. The three atolls demonstrated their skills in turn, dancing and singing, getting louder and louder, with the tin box being beaten faster and faster. One could perceive the dancers getting into a trance-like state, as the music continued. Our group chose to sing a song that they had written themselves. It was rather derogatory as regards the musical ability of the others (or so we were led to believe). They seemed to have the ability to take the micky out of each other. Needless to say, our team won hands down. That's if there was a competition in the first place. Sue said afterwards "That was just magic." We had been so lucky to witness the ceremony. It only happens once every three years, and, had it not been for the fact that the *Faipule* of our atoll was to be made overall Chief, we would not have had the opportunity. The generator kept running until the festivities had finished and so also did the batteries in our video camera. We were confident that we had some good video. We took the boat back to the bungalow, tired but happy.

The happiness was not to last. On returning home, we found that someone had broken into the house, gone through our cases, even opening up our camera cases. They had even taken the telephoto lenses out of their individual cases and left everything strewn over the bed. Oddly, the only things which appeared to have been taken were some small batteries, which fitted both our ordinary still camera and our little tape deck. It looked as if they may have been playing 'doctors' as well. A sphygmomanometer was lying on the sink draining board.

After a little amateur sleuthing, Sue quickly discovered how the break in had been effected; they had wriggled under the storm curtain and then slit the fly screen, pushed out the slats of glass from the louvres and crawled in. Presumably it had been children. As only the batteries had been taken and nothing had been wantonly destroyed, it seemed that the whole exploit had been motivated by curiosity. Sue didn't know what to worry about first, her toes, which had broken out in a weird rash, or the break-in. And I didn't know what to worry about first, Sue's toes, or the fact that so little had been stolen.

Our police officer had captured the culprits in less than four hours. They had been seen by the wood carver, who lived next door to us. He used to sit all day at his carving and he was such a big man that he rarely moved away from his *fale*. There was to be no suspended sentence for them. A week or so later the court was convened; the Elders sat in judgement; and the parents and the rest of the atoll crowded in to the Meeting House. Everyone was there to witness the shame of the children and their parents. That they should have done this to the Doctor and his wife, who were the honoured guests of the atoll, was really to bring disgrace upon the island and its people. We heard that one of the culprits had been the son of a teacher, but we never found out which one. We had not been present at the court hearing and never learned what the punishment was. Almost certainly the shame and loss of face would have been worse than any more tangible penalty. To our knowledge, nothing like it ever occurred again.

On the way to his boat John called in to see us and have a chat. This was unusual. He had previously had to remain on the boat on the open sea, as he had been unable to moor it securely. The mooring had been destroyed by the late lamented Queen Salamasina, the big boat that used to make eight trips a year from Samoa to Tokelau, when money was available. However, it was now safe for him to leave the boat untended, as he had been able to fashion a heavy sea anchor out of something he found on the Atafu Atoll. He was confident that it would hold anything. Fakaofo was a continuous coral reef and, although the land area consisted of a number of individual islands, there was no way for a large boat to get across the reef into the lagoon. Therefore small canoes and inflatables stayed inside the lagoon, while any larger boats had to remain outside the atoll.

John had brought some beer and lots of village gossip; after all, he and his family lived in the middle of the village and his wife, Neta, was well connected. Most of the gossip related to Sue and me. The villagers and the Elders were very favourably disposed towards us and appreciated all we had done and were continuing to do. Of course, Eeoh was still demanding that everything should be done through him, especially any requests for material for repairing the hospital. One had to wonder why this particular aspect should be of such interest to him.

I related to John the recent events, as tactfully as I could, bearing in mind that Neta's father was a respected Elder. I explained how all our attempts to get action through official channels had been thwarted and how, in frustration, we had eventually resorted to broadcasting our complaints direct to Apia. We felt it essential they should be made aware of the condition of the hospital and our reasons for requesting materials to repair it. And at least the strategy had worked, even if it had meant treading on people's toes. We had received the material, or some of it! Whilst we personally had nothing to gain, it was clear that someone else had benefited. Comparison of the bills of lading with the materials actually delivered showed major discrepancies…… but that was another story!

John had heard about the letter I had received from the E.O., but did not know the full details as he had been sailing between the atolls during the relevant period. He was interested to hear how the E.O. had lied at the meeting and had traduced us with his own purported translation of the letter.

After John's departure, we received a visit from the *Faipule*. He wanted to have another look at the original letter. He stayed for two hours and, when he left, he took the letter with him. I was not really quite sure of the purpose of his visit. There seemed to be something going on concerning the two Staff Nurses. The first, Gimaima, was clearly a fraud, but she was married to Eeoh, which put her high up in the hierarchy. Whereas most Tokelauan women had no say and were not even allowed to hold opinions, Gimaima, by her marriage, was clearly in a position of power. Tocina was in a similar position and these two together could do almost as they pleased. I had no illusions that anything we had done would change the *status quo*. Although the islanders wished us to stay, and were very distressed at our imminent departure, we could not delude ourselves into thinking that we would not become more and more isolated, with no real control of the medical service, nor of our own lives either. All those people in authority would be happy to see the back of us. They perceived us as threatening their control. We could imagine just how Dr. Tyo must have felt, totally alone and with no one in whom to confide. At least Sue and I had each other.

At least we realised that there were things going on which we did not understand. I had a nasty feeling that there was a subtle power shift underway on Tokelau and that the three *Faipule* were completely unaware of it. I suspected that the busy Bs, Messrs Balani and Bileti, had been delegated by the New Zealand authorities to sort out the financial drain caused by the 1,500 inhabitants of Tokelau and to resolve their inter-island squabbles.

Just as no one seemed to have any written qualifications, so there appeared to be no published rules or regulations, or, if there were, they were kept very well concealed. Everything had always been ruled by custom and communicated by word of mouth, and this continued to be the case.

Ministering to the Sick

The next day, the women of our island were queuing up for the school boat; the three *Faipule* were still on the atoll and there was to be another meeting. To most of the people, this meant that there would be more feasting; hence the enthusiasm to get on the school boat. We were also invited to attend, by Mr. Balani, who indicated that ties and jackets would again be expected. We did go over to the main island, but not to attend the meeting. The temperature already seemed to be about boiling point and we did not fancy spending the day so overdressed. We preferred to hold our regular clinic and to visit a few patients. Fortunately the wind was beginning to rise, which presaged rain. Sure enough, by the time we reached the other island it was raining heavily. Our practice of visiting the sick in their own homes was an innovation which had been warmly welcomed, particularly by the elderly and the bed-ridden. This hands-on method of healthcare may have fallen out of fashion, but it was nevertheless greatly appreciated on the atoll. For the Doctor to place a child on his knee was something they had never seen before. The look of pleasure and pride on the mothers' faces had to be seen, and the kids thought it wonderful. It was just unknown for patients to be touched or physically examined.

I did the clinic with Leki. One of the patients was a little boy with what I suspected to be a thyroglossal cyst. I made a note to get him transferred to the mainland for further examination and treatment.

As we made our rounds, I received a message, would we like to have lunch with the Elders? Perhaps they thought that they might need a home visit in the future. Before our arrival on Tokelau, anyone who had wanted to see the Doctor had to find his way to the hospital – even if that entailed a trip across the lagoon lying on an old door! Perhaps the Elders were finally appreciating the changes which we had introduced.

We were met at the Meeting House by our *Faipule*, who returned my letter, much to my relief. We went into lunch together.

Dr. Zona shared with me the responsibility for running the hospital, even though he was officially retired. He informed me that he and his brother, Dr. Liutta, the Medical Director, had decided to allow one of our nurses, Margarita, to return to her home atoll. Her mother had been brought to our atoll after Margarita had tearfully confided to us that she was dying of cancer. We had diagnosed her as a case of severe diabetes and had managed, with some difficulty, to stabilise her condition. Knowing that background and all our nursing problems, it seemed inconceivable that Dr. Zona should have conspired in a decision to give one of our better nurses a month's leave. To rub salt into the wound, they offered me another health visitor. I had learned that Gimaima, who had been appointed Staff Nurse, was by qualification a health visitor. Having suspended her for incompetence, I was now being offered another of the same. I would be left with a complement of just two real nurses, including Tocina, whose attendance could never be guaranteed.

On returning to the boat we were stopped by one of our lads in blue, well, not exactly one of ours, as he had come with the delegation from one of the other atolls for the installation of the new Chief. He was a good six feet six and very smart in his dress uniform. He drew himself up to his full height and saluted, "Permission to speak, Sir?" "Oh, for God's sake," I said to Sue, "have we parked on double yellow lines again?" At this, his face broke into a gorgeous beam.

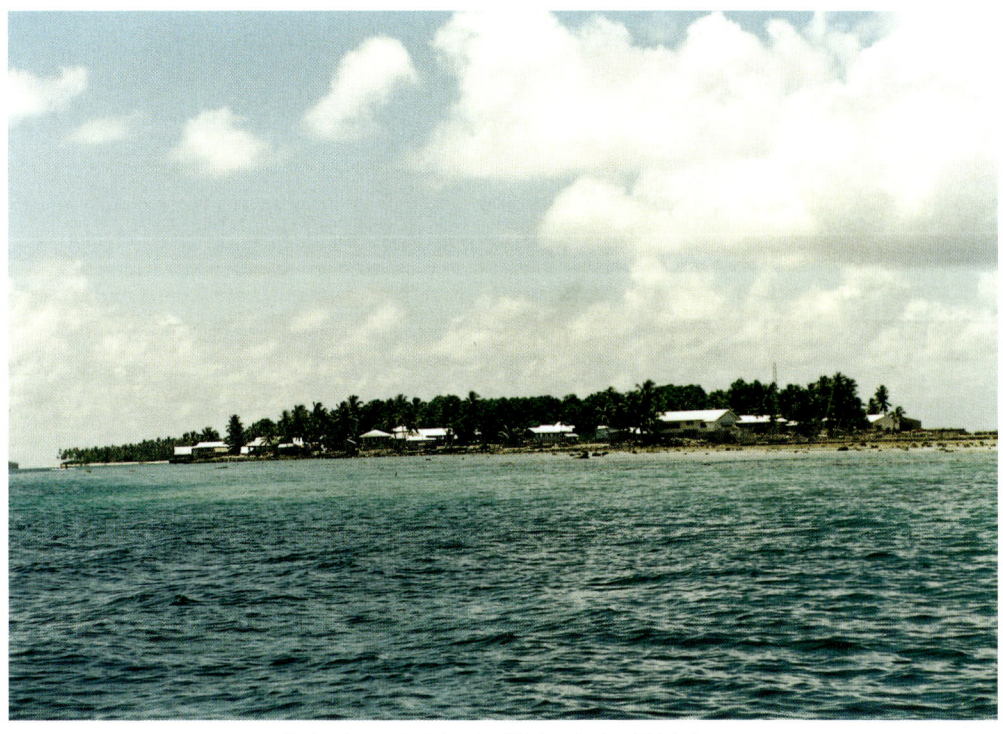

Fale, the main island of Fakaofo Atoll Tokelau.

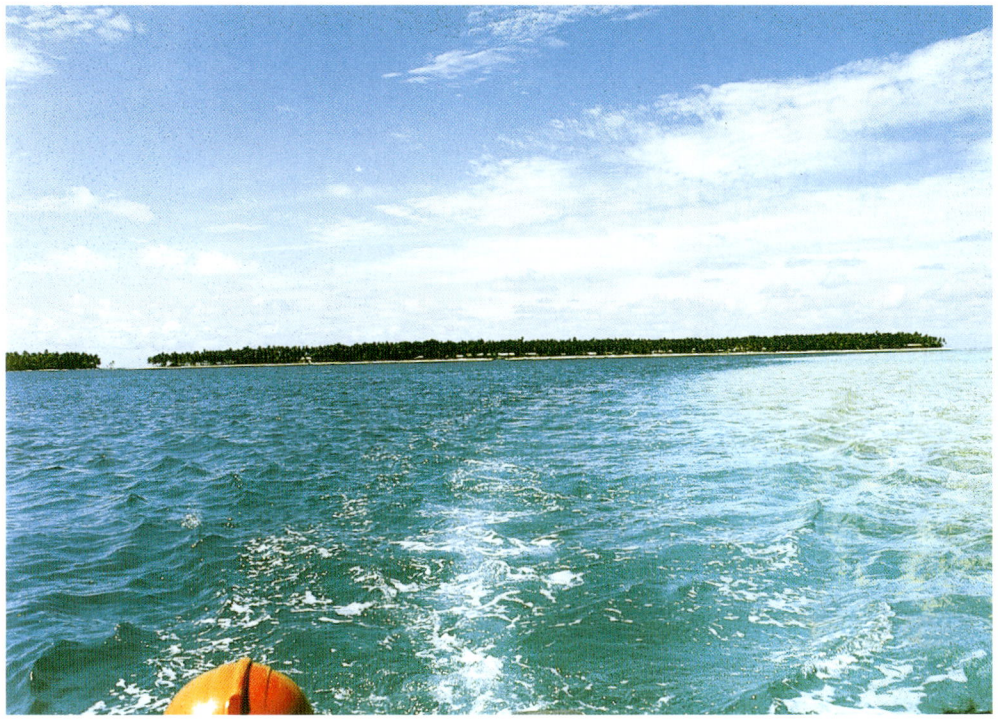

Fenna Fala, our island, the site of the school and hospital.

FAKAOFO

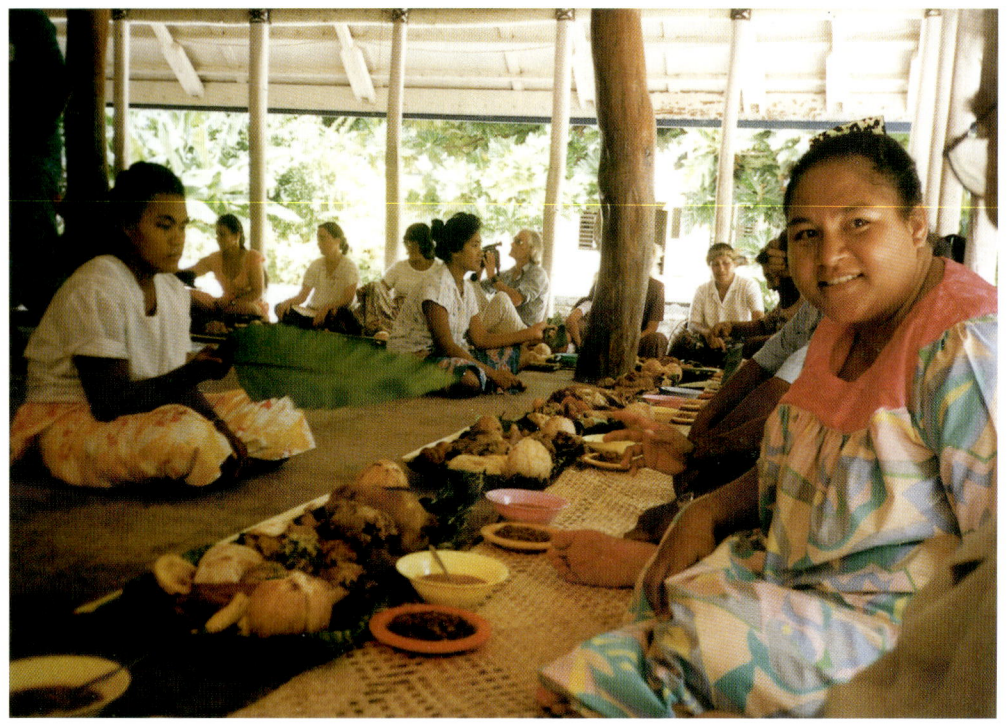

Welcoming feast in the Meeting House.

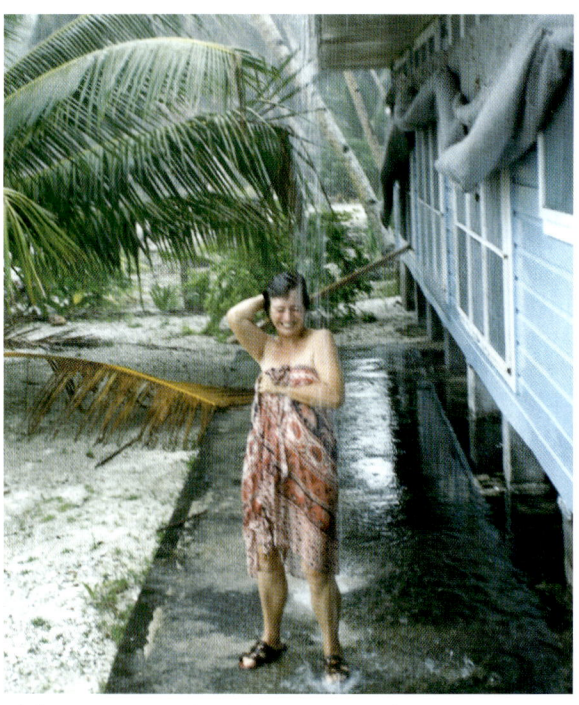

*A tropical downpour, Sue takes advantage of the broken gutter for a shower.
On the right, the storm curtain over the window.*

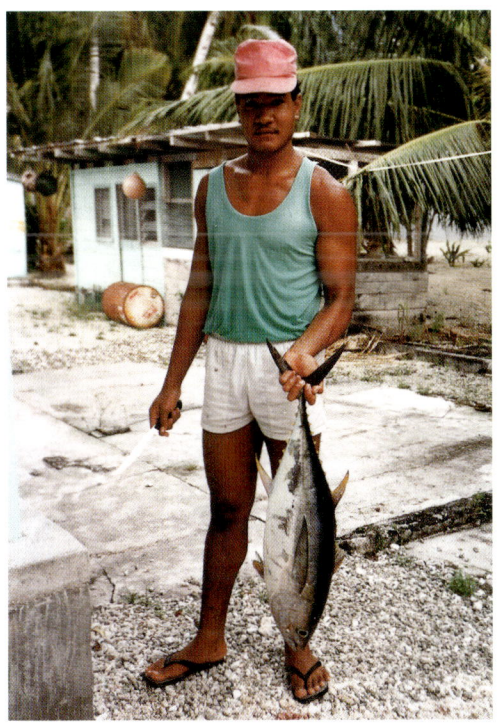
Our hospital boat lad, bringing us another fish.

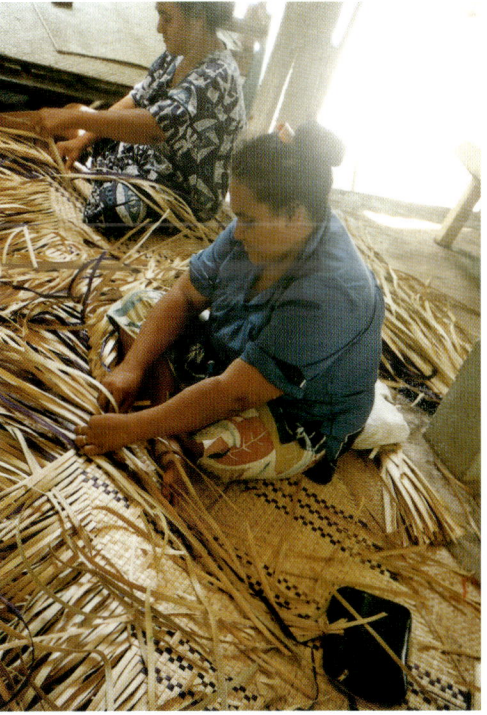
All women make sleeping mats for their homes.

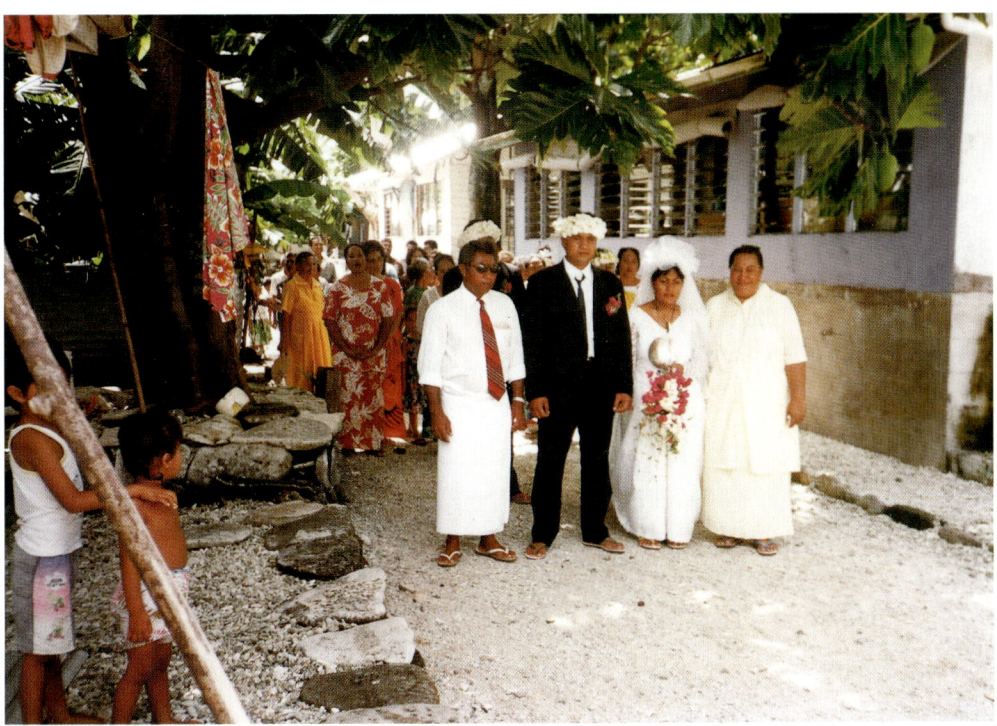
Bride and Groom walking around the island after their wedding, with R.C. Priest and his wife either side.

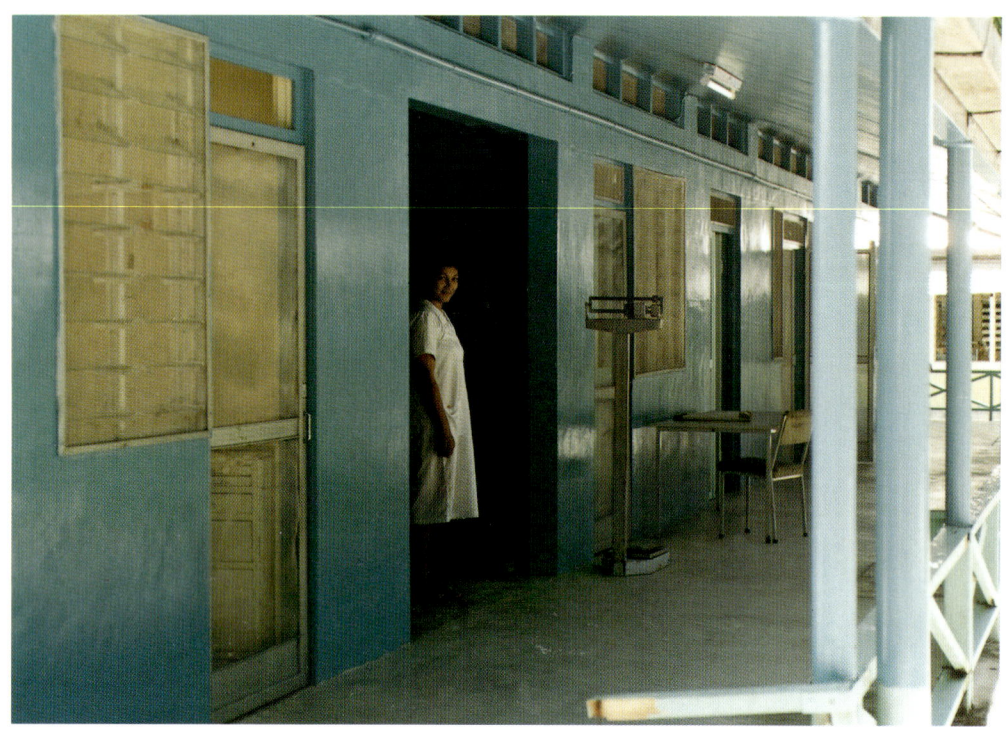
Nurse Leki in the entrance to the hospital on Fenna Fala.

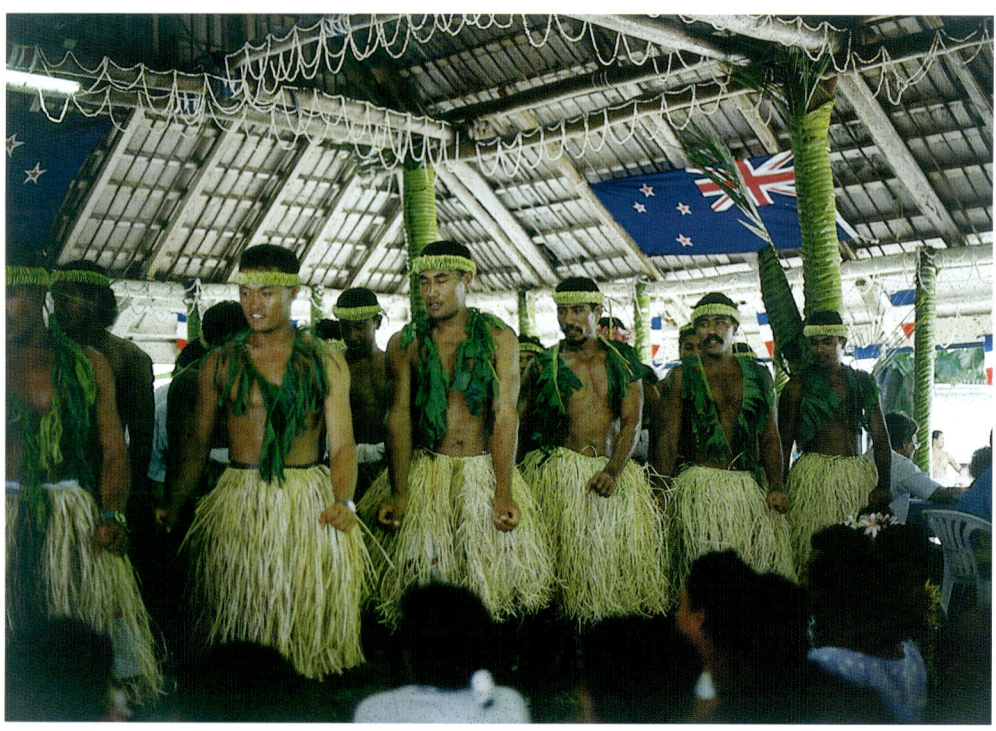
Dancing at the festival of our Chief being made Chief of all three atolls.

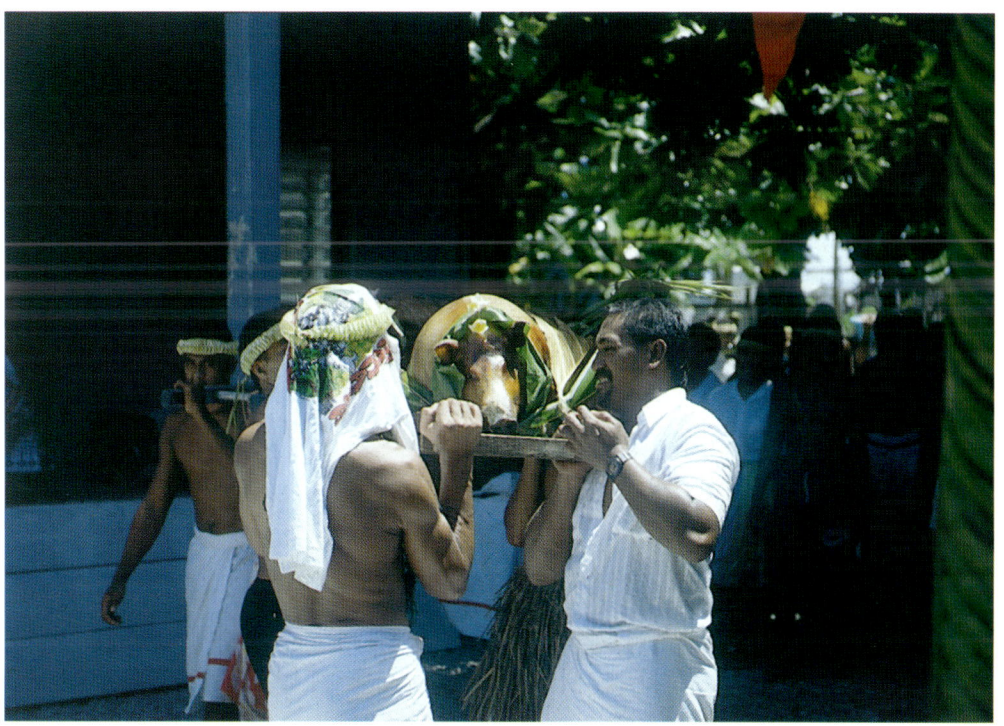

The roasted pig in procession around the island before being eaten by the dignitaries.

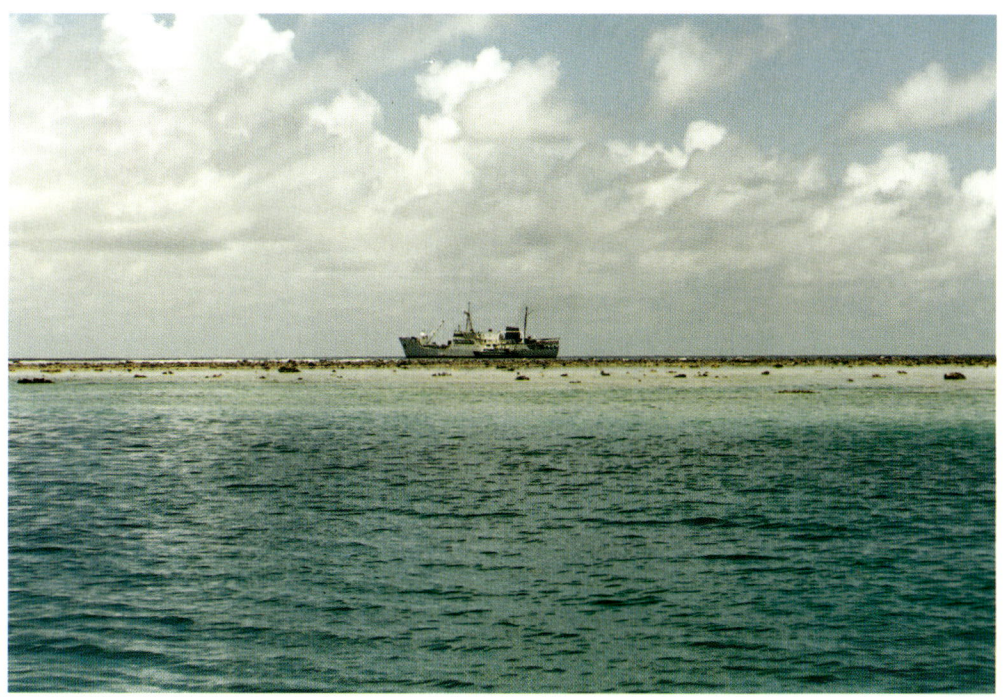

The Cape Don anchored off Fakaofo Atoll on the seaward side of the reef beside the much smaller M.V. Tutolo.

SAVAII

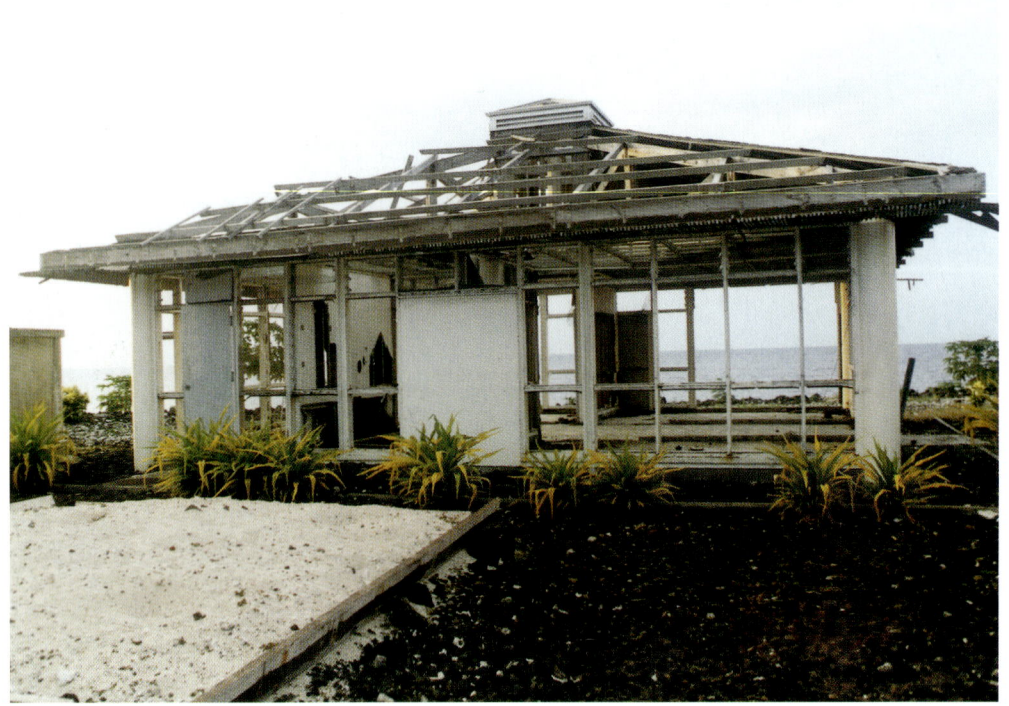

The remains of the Doctor's house at Sataua Hospital after the last hurricane.

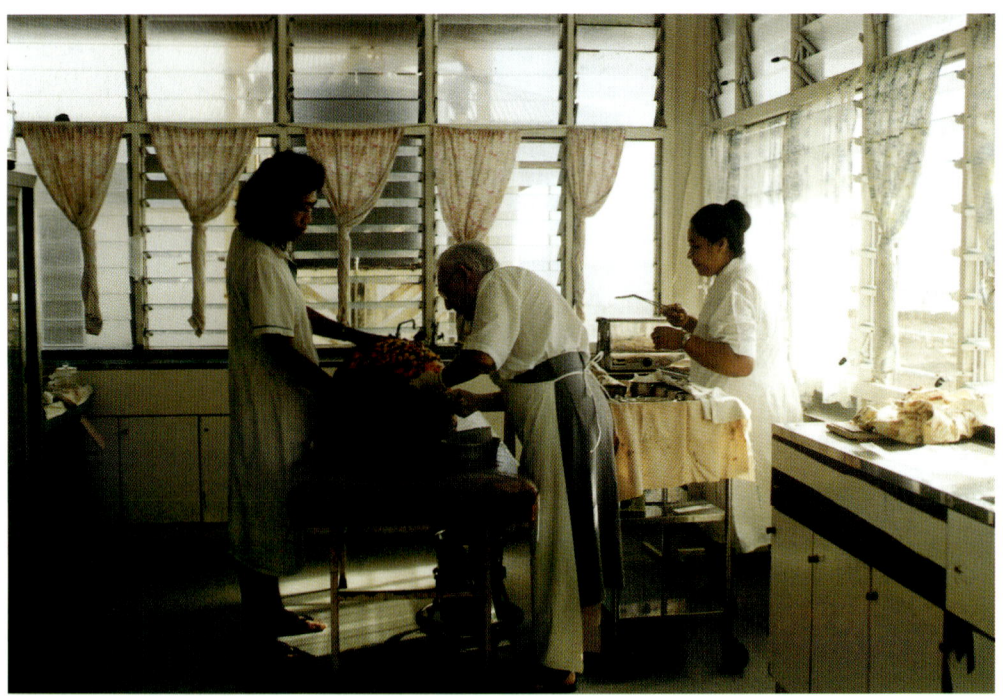

In the operating room of the hospital at Sataua. Dr. Max with Alua on the right, during a minor operation.

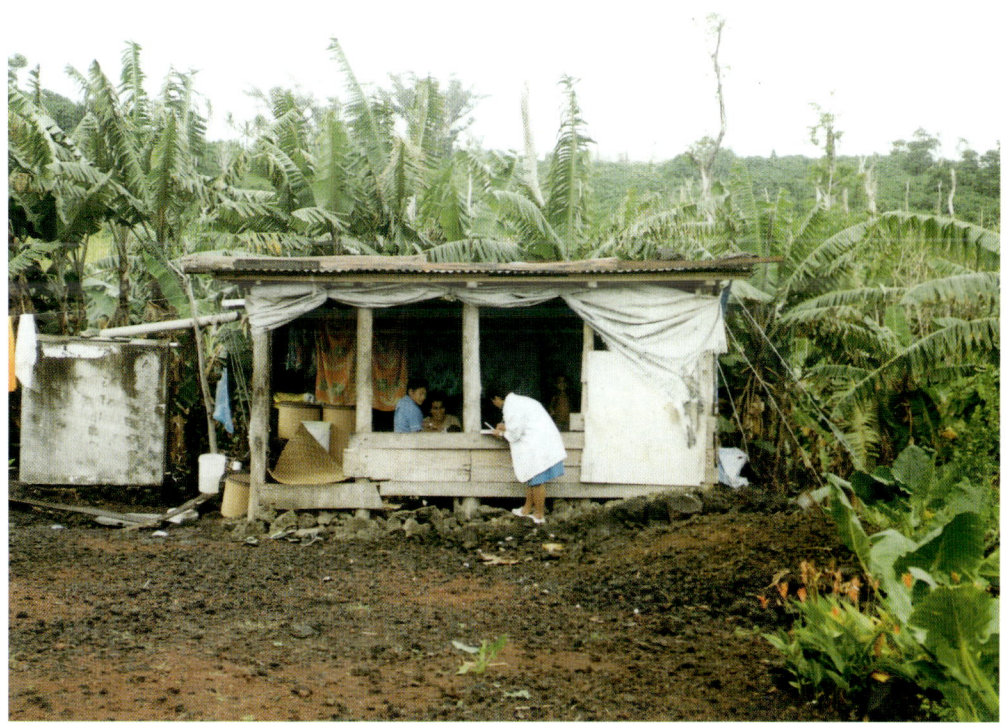
Recording the immunisation at the home of a new baby on a visit to the plantations with nurse Toy Eva.

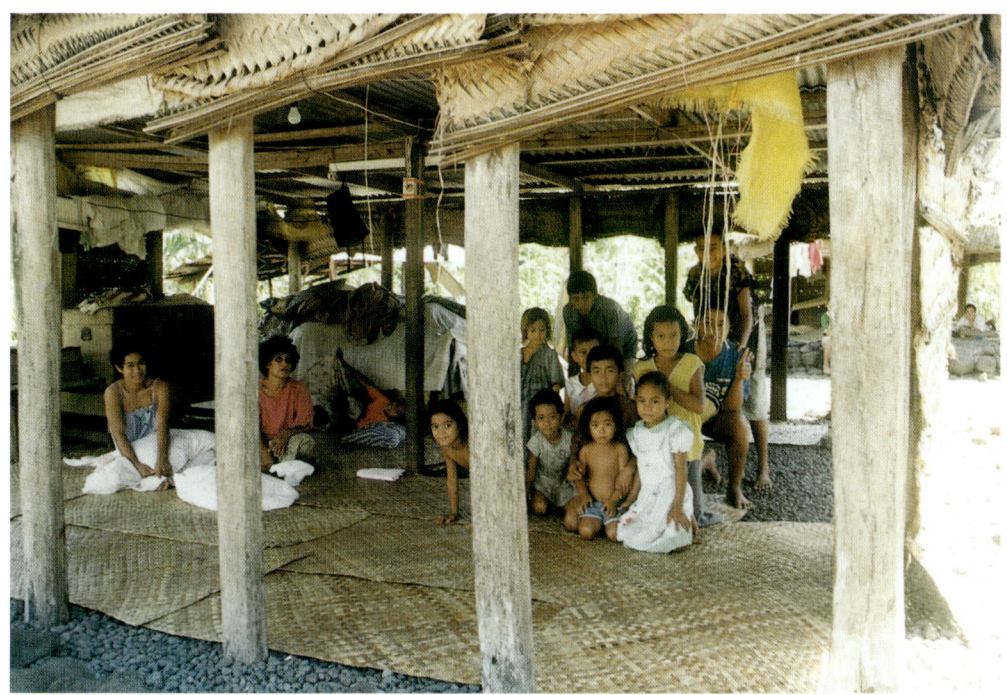
Dr. Max making a house call on the way back from Manase and taking patient on the left back with him to Sataua hospital.

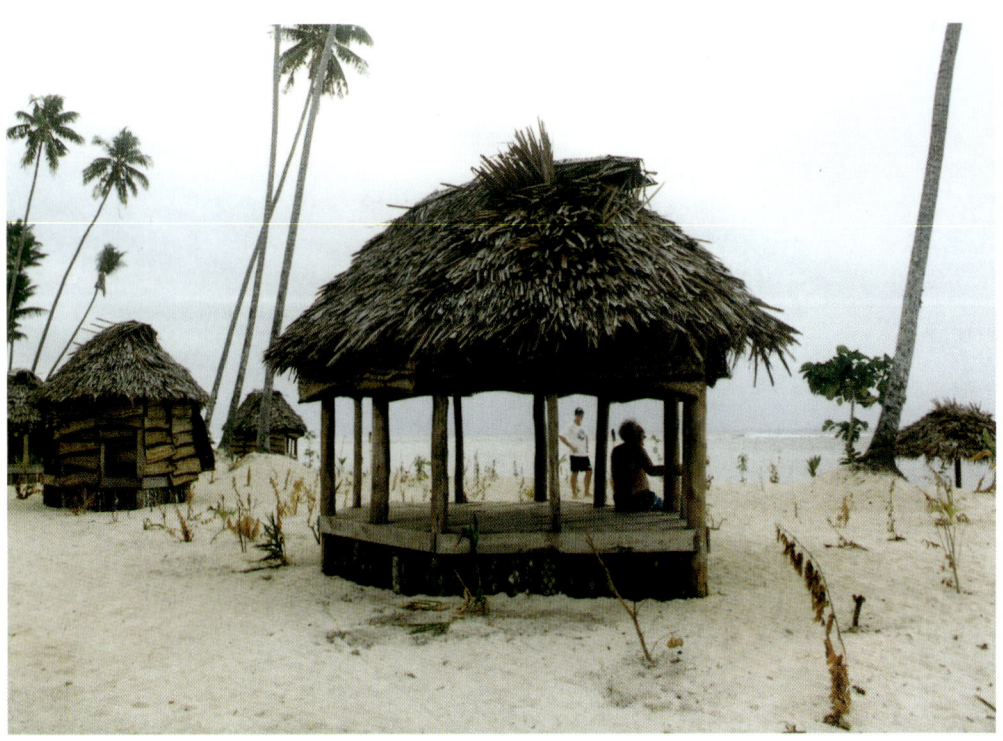

The beach Fales at Manase on the week-end of the Hash Harriers get together.

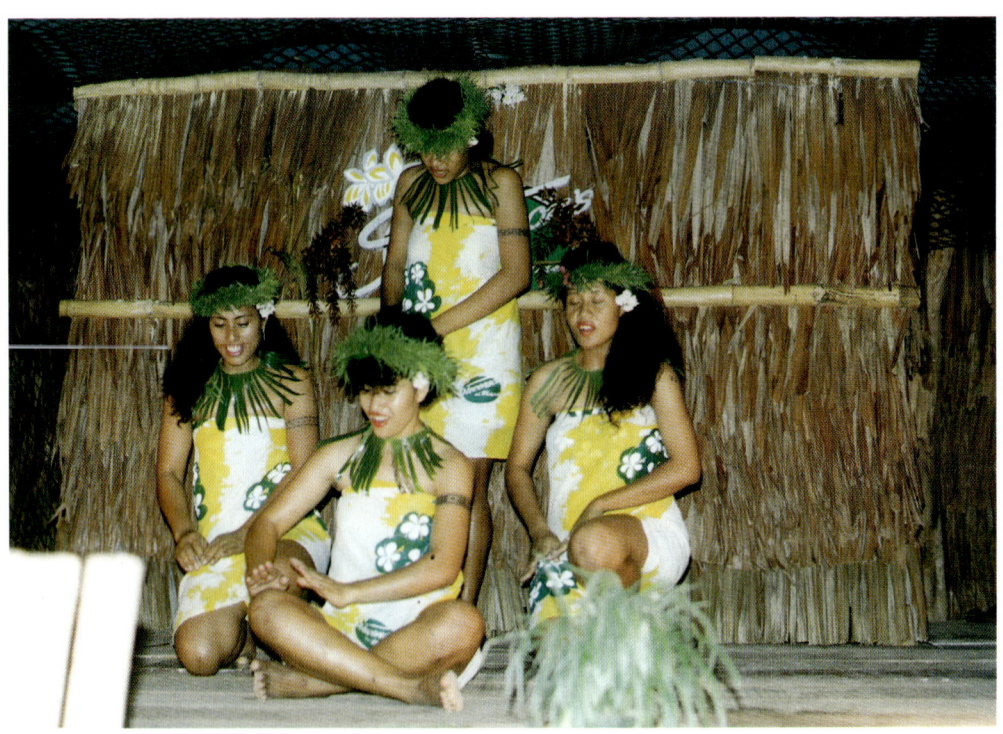

The Manase group entertaining us during the evening meal.

"You like it here? You like to try it my home?" We were being propositioned again! Once again we were being tempted with an alternative. We had a moment of doubt and uncertainty. There was no reason why we should not, after our holiday in New Zealand, return to one of the other atolls and have an easy time for three months. Sue was adamant; "No," she said, " we would be faced with the same problems all over again." So we thanked the officer nicely, and said that we had promised the people of Faka that we would stay with them.

What an interesting day it turned out to be; we had not even reached home when the *Faipule* from Nukunonu and his wife approached us. There were the usual formalities and small talk, and then – would we like to think about coming to their atoll and doing for them what we had done for Fakaofo? We didn't know whether to laugh or cry about it all.

We returned to the hospital, where there were a number of visitors. We were by this time giving conducted tours round the hospital. Even the patients were beginning to join in and talk with the visitors. It was all very jolly; it was clear that we had made a hit.

We had survived another day, but the night was bad, I couldn't sleep and kept going over and over in my mind my address to the Elders at the lunch earlier in the day.

I was still feeling very hurt. I remembered starting off by telling them that if anyone asked me if we had enjoyed our stay on Fakaofo, I would reply that yes, we had. We had been robbed and we had been insulted, not only verbally, but also in writing. I continued, "You have been informed that there have been arguments between the E.O., his wife and us. It is he who has written a most insulting letter to us. It is he who has lied to you concerning the translation of that letter, so that you did not know what he had really written. I suspended his wife because of her lack of even basic nursing knowledge and her insulting behaviour to her patients. As for your hospital, we have done in 12 weeks what others have failed to do in 15 years. Ask your E.O. what he has done except try to stop us every day in every way. I ask you to go out there and ask your people, ask your women, especially those with young babies, if they are happy with the things that we have done. Some of you Elders have been lied to here, under this very roof. To think that this E.O. is also a lay preacher, it really makes you wonder. We did not travel half way round the world to be lied to. Go outside and ask the people if they trust us. Go outside and ask your women and the old folk if what we have done was for our benefit or for their benefit. We are leaving!!!..."

I always felt better after this sort of exercise and, having cleared my mind and my conscience, I fell asleep.

There were just a few patients to see when I entered the hospital the next morning. It was Monday 31st January 1994. It seemed that I had recently been seeing more visitors than patients and this day was no exception. Having deflected the approach by the *Faipule* of Nukunonu, I was surprised to see the *Faipule* of the third atoll, Atafu, waiting to see me. How would we like to go up to his atoll? By now we had made up our minds and were completely resolved in our decision. We would leave Tokelau and would not return to any of its atolls. I would not compromise in what I believed to be the right way of doing things. There was still much to do in the short time we had left and it seemed pointless to continue arguing for improvements, which would not happen. I courteously declined the *Faipule's* offer and turned my attention to the waiting patients.

Regardless of our battles with officialdom, the majority of the islanders continued to be extremely hospitable to us. Every day we found provisions left at our door: on one day it would be fresh fish; on another chicken pieces, or a couple of eggs (not knowing the provenance of the eggs did cause us a moment's hesitation before eating them); there was even a leaf basket filled with fresh coconuts. We had not seen so much food since arriving on the island.

Sue and I did our rounds of the hospital. We had finished the stocktaking, noting the many items we had which we could not use and the lack of most of the drugs and equipment needed to run an efficient hospital service. We had managed to make the best use of the little we had, but we doubted whether the system would survive for a month after our departure. The half-hearted nature of the maintenance work made us wonder if the painting and decorating would ever be completed. We would leave with sorrow the people of the atoll whom we realised we would, in a sense, be abandoning. They deserved so much more; more opportunities, more facilities and more hopes for the future. More frustratingly we knew that, with a little organisation and conscientious application by the officials in charge, they could actually have had so much more. It was very difficult for a lone *papalagi* to make a real impact in a society where customs and rank were so entrenched. However, we would leave with no regrets for what we had, or had not, done. We knew that we had done our best.

When I awoke the next morning, Sue told me that I had slept through a *Donner und Blitzen* night, a real tropical storm, with thunder and lightning to awaken the dead. The fact that I had slept through it suggested that life in a tropical paradise was rather more exhausting than it was generally cracked up to be. In view of this observation, I was surprised and delighted to note that, since arriving on Tokelau, my blood pressure had remained normal, without me having to take any of my usual tablets. The change could not be attributed to workload or stress, as I was experiencing plenty of both, so I could only put it down to the tropical climate, or the food. Certainly the virtually meat-free diet was quite different from that which I would normally have eaten at home.

Of course, the introduction of western foods had made an impact on the lifestyles of the local population and in general it was an adverse one. Beer, Coca-Cola, cigarettes, sugar and tinned foods had all contributed to a general deterioration in health standards. One only had to look at the dreadful life statistics of the Tokelauan people since the arrival of the Europeans; the widespread tooth decay, the high level of diabetes, where there had been none previously, and the soaring numbers of people suffering from high blood pressure. It put me in mind of the plagues visited upon the poor old Egyptians.

Having dealt with the short queue of patients waiting at the hospital, I was just settling down for a quite day, when I was surprised to receive a most unexpected patient. I was used to old Dr. Zona popping in for a chat, but not for emergency medical treatment. It transpired that, some days previously, he had been fooling about with one of his grandchildren when one of them trod on an old shaving mirror, which happened to have been lying on the sleeping mat. Zona had then paddled through the pieces of broken mirror in his bare feet. Like all doctors, he had been reluctant to seek medical attention, so by now infection had set in.

I raided the medical supplies in the dental store, knowing that their anaesthetics were relatively fresh, only three years past their sell-by dates! We pumped him full of antibiotics, but I knew that I would have to open up the foot to remove the slivers of glass. As previously explained, most of the surgical instruments in the hospital were rusty and unusable, but fortunately I had my own set, which had been donated by our local hospital in Yorkshire. Sue had done a great job to keep them in prime condition. They were some fine instruments.

It took me over an hour, by which time I had removed at least five pieces of glass. I felt sure that there were more, but could not find them. With any luck, Mother Nature would push them to the surface in due course. Dr. Zona had endured the pain without a murmur, but it would not have been fair to continue probing inside his foot. I just hoped that, with the incision closed up and the foot carefully strapped, my efforts would have made his foot feel easier. Since arriving on the atoll, I had suffered considerable discomfort with my own feet. However, some days earlier, because the water from our tap was becoming increasingly salty, I had decided to avoid drinking it and to stick to nothing but coconut milk. Since then, my previously swollen feet had reduced back to their normal size. The worrying thing was that the hospital patients were being given the same water that came from our tap.

It was in the early hours of the following morning, when we were roused from our beds to deal with a patient brought over from the other island. It must be the same the world over, this tendency to wait until the middle of the night to bring in the most chronic cases. This one was a 'beauty', a case of diabetes, aggravated by several large, dirty ulcers on top of the patient's foot. I would need to clean them up straight away. I was surprised that I had not seen the woman before.

I was pleased to find Sue by my side. With no nursing staff awake, it was wonderful to have Sue to assist me. I knew that she would do it well. We would clean up the wounds and make the patient comfortable. The task of cutting out the dead flesh and sorting out the diabetes could wait until morning. What really annoyed me was that this must have been one of Gimaima's patients. Why had she not referred her to me earlier?

Despite the disrupted night's rest, I needed to get into the hospital in the morning, as I had a couple of patients requiring suction clearance of their ears. As usual, the hospital was lacking the basic equipment needed for this procedure, so I had cobbled together a bit of apparatus of my own. I had connected a spinal needle, cut down to a suitable length, and connected that to a suction pump. The needle was just the right size to fit through the aperture of the auriscope, so, after flushing out the ear, I was able to clean out the ear with the suction pump whilst at the same time seeing exactly what was happening. It may not have been standard equipment, but it worked and I was very pleased with the outcome.

Meanwhile Sue was manning the dispensary. There was quite a queue – and they all wanted Dramamine tablets. We found it strange that these island people, whose ancestors had all been seafarers, should suffer so greatly from seasickness the moment they got near an ocean-going boat. Everyone knew that the boat was due within the next few days, so they wanted to stock up with seasickness pills before it arrived. No one new exactly when to expect the boat, but then its schedule was always based on 'Tokelauan time'. It was 'par for the course'.

One couple awaiting the arrival of the boat were the *Faipule* of Atafu and his wife. Having been rebuffed on their approach to me two days earlier, they had returned to the hospital, not to try further persuasion, but to request that I give them a general examination. With the demise of Dr. Tyo, they no longer had any qualified medical service on their atoll, so they understandably wished to make the most of their opportunity before they left Fakaofo. From what we were hearing, conditions on our atoll, limited as they were, were far better than on Atafu and Nukunonu.

Just as we had bade farewell to the *Faipule*, I saw Soshe's parents approaching. They had been fishing and were bringing a big bonito and a parrot fish, caught in the lagoon. Much as we felt heartily sick at the sight of fish, we had to recognise that it was a most generous gift.

Back in the hospital ward I was anxious to see how our diabetic patient was progressing. Her foot certainly looked bad and I decided to use Cloxacillin on her. As with all of our drugs, it was out of date. It was a gamble, but usually I got away with it. This time I didn't and I nearly lost, or at least, the patient nearly lost. There was a massive reaction to the injection and she collapsed. It took us two hours to get her back and stable. Meanwhile her husband, who was sleeping on the floor beside her bed, did not awaken, in spite of everything that was going on next to him.

The following morning, Sue got up at 5.00 a.m. to check the patient's blood sugar level and, upon her return, whispered to me that the husband had still not moved. I asked her if she had checked that he was still alive. She said she hadn't, but thought that his loud snoring was probably a good indication.

I had been trying to deal with one particularly bad case of bronchitis and it was giving me real cause for concern. The reason was that the patient was myself. My temperature was up and the sputum was a thick green colour. I was going to have to stay in bed unless I really had to get up. I also had to decide which of my suspect drugs I could safely use on myself. "Physician heal thyself." I wrote up my log for the previous 24 hours and retired to my bed. As I dropped off to sleep, I recalled something John had told me when he had called in almost a week before. It was something, which he had picked up on his radio. As previously mentioned, John had the best receiver in the area and was invariably ahead of everyone else in getting the news. Incidentally, I have heard that, at a later date, the Elders tried to confiscate John's radio, as they found it very inconvenient that he always knew what was going on before they did.

However, the events which John related had apparently occurred in Western Samoa.

In a remote village, one of the villagers had worked hard to better his family, a most unusual thing in these little villages, where the people all live in the same abject poverty. In general, the population is just one big extended family, and in theory everything belongs to everyone. This would be fine, except that they often forget to return anything that they have borrowed. It's much simpler that way. Anyway, this villager decided to open a small store – and by dint of tight financial management, he made it pay. Later, realising that one of the difficulties of the village was that it was cut off from Apia, the capital and only major town, with not even a bus connection, he decided it needed some public transport. He bought himself a clapped out old bus, and set up a one-man bus service, not only into Apia, but also to other villages around.

That was where the trouble started. It seems that the rest of the villagers felt that he should share his new wealth with them, and when he explained that he and his family had built up the business without any help, and that it rightfully belonged only to his family, they took strong exception to the idea. They shot him and severely injured the other members of his family. Then, just to show how wrong he had been, the villagers burnt down the store and set fire to the bus. The surviving members of the family were driven out of the village.

Word spread around the island of Western Samoa. The police knew of it and it was even reported in the local newspaper. Nevertheless, it took the central government several weeks to react. After all, Government House was more than 20 miles from the village. However, the officials did eventually get to hear of it and, as the villagers' action was a direct snub to the government, they had to act.

The case came to court, with the villagers claiming that the village Elders were the people who made the local rules and not these upstarts in the Parliament. It was a lawyer's dream and the case dragged on for months, while the accused Elders tried to enlist the support of other villages. However, as most of them were dependent upon central government for subsidies and the payment of dole money, support was half-hearted and the government was bound to win in the end. This virtual declaration of independence could not be allowed to succeed, or other villagers would undoubtedly follow suit.

The ringleaders were identified and the offenders were all given hefty sentences. The jail had to be revamped for them, it not having been used for many years. The families had to take food to the prisoners every day, as the jail couldn't provide any, and all the prisoners were allowed to go home to their villages for the weekends, as the prison was only staffed from Friday to Monday.

Everyone was satisfied. The government had shown that it made the rules, and the village Elders were allowed to retain a certain amount of their local autonomy. It was a good story, and, according to John, it was all true.

Sue had been looking for some of my white shirts. We still more or less lived out of our suitcases. At least this kept the larger cockroaches out of our clothing. It would seem impossible to lose shirts, while they were being stored in a suitcase, but Sue could not find them; it was one more South Pacific mystery.

It must have been the thought of all that spare space in the suitcase that prompted Sue to go across to have a chat with the wood carver. Using Leki as her interpreter, Sue asked whether he could make her a bowl. After sending his son to scour the island for a suitable piece of wood, he had to admit defeat. All he could offer was a model of the traditional boats used on the atolls. He made a beautiful job of them and had a ready market back in Apia, but it was sad that lack of materials restricted him to this single subject.

I was still feeling ill, but dragged myself out of bed to deal with another case referred to us from the main island. Once again it was a woman suffering from diabetes and someone whom I had never seen before. This must have been another of Gimaima's patients. It was clear that Leki was tracking them down and sending them across to us for treatment. I wondered how many more of the islanders were diabetic? The problem was compounded by the wrong food; they didn't seem to understand what they needed to eat, and what was dangerous for them. Each morning the women made a fire, put whatever they had available in the pot, and cooked it for most of the day; it could be taro, green bananas, or breadfruit. Unfortunately much of the diet was based on root vegetables and other foods high in carbohydrates, which turned into sugar and exacerbated the diabetes.

I looked in to check on the diabetic whom we had so nearly lost the other night. She was doing very well, although I could see that it would take some time for her ulcers to heal properly. I would have to check what we had available in the drug cupboard.

Sue was taking over more and more of the administration of the hospital. While I checked on the patients, she was busy doing the sterilising. Everything was put into the steriliser and brought to the boil. It came out a beautiful yellow colour, much more impressive than the dirty white, which we used to get.

Sue came back from a visit to the radio shack. More aggro! Although I was supposed to be in charge of everything to do with the hospital, they insisted on interfering. They called it negotiating, which meant that I should agree to observe any directions from Apia, regardless of the needs or desires of the people in Tokelau. However, one had to remember all the time that the people at the top of the tree in the Tokelauan Office in Apia, were all related to the top families residing in the Tokelauan atolls. The important news from the radio shack was the information that Steve had not cancelled the order for the refrigerator. We could not understand why he had ignored our request. The other piece of information was that Steve and Dr. Liutta were coming to Tokelau on the next boat. It seemed that the officials in Apia were all in a flat spin. They wanted to talk to us. It was a pity that they had left it too late!

There was a cool breeze blowing. It would almost certainly be followed, in about a quarter of an hour, by a rainstorm. This was almost invariably the case and it was usually a tropical downpour, nice and warm.

Our nurse, Margareta, came over to ask Sue about the sterilising, and yet she was supposed to be one of the fully trained nurses. Sue had made me feel very proud of her; she had coped so wonderfully well and learnt so fast, particularly considering that she had no formal nursing training. Thanks to her natural intelligence and ability, the trained nurses were now coming to her for advice.

In addition to the radio-telephone, there was a tele-printer on the other island. It was intended only for government and official use, but it appeared that almost everyone was using it. In fact, it looked as if we were the only ones not using it. From what we heard, it seemed that much of the traffic concerned us, and most showed us in a favourable light. The islanders were even beginning to use the phrase 'the *papalagi* way'. We could only wait and see if anything came of it. The main thing was it lightened the atmosphere, and Sue was certainly pleased with the feedback she was getting. Her source was the radio operator, who was, of course, Yanetta's husband.

I was still suffering from a really bad chest. In addition to this, Sue was insisting on taking my blood pressure regularly, as it was beginning to go back up. I thought I would probably have to go back on treatment. Never mind, it had been a nice break.

As I was still feeling 'under the weather', Sue was continuing to take the lead rôle in running the hospital. Still, the nurses seemed content with the situation and certainly the patients were happy. The only ones to complain were those who did not actually do any work, like the E.O. He was most upset with Sue. Ideally he would have liked her out. That would not have pleased the nursing staff. They were only too happy for Sue to continue doing the dirty work. Who cleaned down the walls in preparation for Gred to throw on his new paint? Sue. Who changed the patients' dirty dressing every few hours? Sue. Who was treating the infected ulcers with antibiotics? Who else? Of course, it was Sue.

And the main thing was, she was winning. In particular, those awful ulcers were responding to her treatment.

Of course, when the boat arrived in three weeks time (or so it was rumoured), everything would change. What order we had brought would be replaced once again by chaos and incompetence. Margareta and her mother would return to their own atoll. Leki would probably rebel against the idiocy of it all and would take herself and her family back to New Zealand. I knew from Dr. Zona that they had relatives living in the North Island. In fact, there was a large group of people from Tokelau living around Auckland. It was everyone's dream to be able to go there. Unfortunately very few would be able to realise that dream.

As the week progressed, I felt increasingly recovered from my bronchitis and got more involved in the running of the hospital. By the end of the first day back at work, I was beginning to wonder whether that had been a wise decision. Firstly, Neta had asked me to help her to extract a back tooth of one of her dental patients. Very foolishly I agreed to help her. Up until that time, I had been unaware of a fact, apparently known to all dentists; namely that the people in the Pacific have the toughest jaws in the whole world. Neta had already injected the patient with at least twice the normal dose of local anaesthetic and had succeeded in breaking off the tooth more or less flush with the gum. The patient was a brave man, certainly braver than I was. After endeavouring to drill down the side of the tooth to get either a chisel or forceps onto the offending root, I lost my nerve; his jaw was like iron, my grip had gone, my hand was shaking, my nerves were shot; only the patient seemed to be happy. All this time we had had no power and therefore had neither lighting nor suction. I was even having to use the old foot operated drill. We had to admit defeat. We cleaned the patient up and explained that he would need bigger tools than we had in Tokelau. He would have to go on the next boat to Apia and the big hospital. Neta and I were very disappointed at having failed the patient, but he was as happy as Larry, particularly at the prospect of going to Samoa.

On going into the ward, I found one of the nurses taking the scabs off the diabetic patient's leg using her own little pocket penknife. So much for her competence and so much for my attempts at staff training! It hadn't been a good day so far.

I rescued myself, and went off to have a talk with Mr. Bileti, the guy from the T.P.S. (Tokelauan Public Services). He was the new great master. According to the new rules and regulations being promulgated by himself and by Mr. Balani, they were the only persons with the power to hire and or fire anyone. They purported to act in the name of the New Zealand government and it was they who had been instrumental in formulating the very nice letter that I received the other day from the *Faipule*, stressing how grateful they all were for my efforts with regards to the patients and the hospital, but nevertheless informing me that I would have to accept back the two suspended nurses. The letter conveniently omitted to mention the fact that the two nurses were incompetent. However, by this time I knew that it was going to be their problem and not mine; the boat was only one week away.

Despite all the frustrations and disappointments, we still found it difficult to face up to the thought of leaving. Over supper, Sue was actually talking about going up to Atafu, the atoll 100 miles to the north of us. After the unsuccessful approach by the *Faipule*, they had sent down Margareta's brother to try and talk us into going up there to reorganise their hospital. In one respect I suppose it might have been a good idea; a different location, a different challenge. However, on reflection, we decided that we would probably end up with similar problems to those, which we had faced when we first arrived on Fakaofo: better the devil you know… Besides, we liked the people on 'our' atoll. Even more importantly, the people liked us!

The next day I received a visit from Melli's wife. She presented me with a rather dirty wound on her great toe, not an unusual type of injury, as most people do not even wear sandals, and the atolls consist of nothing but sharp coral. Melli himself had got into conversation with Sue. It appeared that the Elders, or at least, some of them, had at last learned the truth about the letter and the mis-translation presented to them. They had challenged the E.O. for an explanation, but the best he could offer was "I don't know why I did it!" Of course Sue knew exactly why he had done it. He had been incited to do it by both his wife Gimaima, and by the Senior Nurse Tocina. They were pathetic; I almost felt sorry for them.

Gred's painting always amazed me. Not satisfied with the gecko, he had now immortalised even more animal life on the walls of the hospital. I supposed it would give future patients something to ponder over, together with the out-of-date calendar and list of telephone numbers, both now covered in a smooth coat of vinyl matt. The loss of the telephone numbers would probably not cause too much inconvenience, as the telephone had not worked since the end of the last war! It would probably be a similar interval of time until the hospital received its next coat of paint.

There was considerable chatter in the wards that night. Somehow they had heard that the boat had been delayed yet again. We learned the news with dismay. Bang went our flight reservations for our holiday to New Zealand. Oh well, there was nothing we could do about it. Win some; lose some! – although the 'lose some' seemed to be in the ascendant.

I always entered the storeroom with some trepidation. One never knew what variety of creepy-crawly would be hiding in the shadows. Still, it was always interesting. There was invariably something new to discover. One day I turned up some very old records of radio traffic. It seemed that, as far back as the 1960s, Dr. Zona had been pleading for essential supplies for the hospital. It was clear that he had been treated with the same scant respect then as now. Even then, he had been trying to get the atoll cleaned up, to get rid of the mosquitoes and flies. The response from Samoa had been just claptrap. Obviously not much had changed in 30 years.

Hidden in the recesses of the storeroom I came across a copy of Zona's contract. It was weird; Tocina was shown as being in charge of the hospital, with Dr. Zona being subordinate to her. I wondered if this was part of the price he paid for his religious views. It probably also explained the rather odd arrangement whereby, whilst he would diagnose the patient's ailment, it was Tocina who would decide whether anything would be done. This gave credence to a story told us by Leki. Apparently Dr. Zona diagnosed a patient as having acute appendicitis. He asked for the theatre to be prepared for an urgent operation, but Tocina overruled him, so that was the end of the matter. The patient died. Of course, that was one more black mark against Dr. Zona.

All this helped explain Leki's vehement dislike of Tocina – and why we got on so well with Leki. We had gone out of our way to help her father and to have him re-integrated into society.

I was having a devil of a job trying to stabilise our non-insulin-dependent diabetics. We had no accurate means of measuring blood sugar levels, as our inadequate little meter had no means of resetting it. The calibration units had been lost in the distant past. No one had explained that these test kits were essential for setting up the meter correctly on a regular basis. I had had no alternative but to set it up by using Sue, Leki and myself as controls, taking our average blood sugar level as 'normal'. It seemed to work, but it would have been nice to have a proper calibration as confirmation. Even with an estimate of blood sugar, it was a real headache to devise a diet for each individual diabetic patient.

As I was pondering this problem, Dr. Zona called in for another little chat. I was pleased to see that his foot had healed and he was walking without discomfort. He had brought a bottle of home-brew with him; clearly we were in for a long session.

It was the same old subject – our future. He said he would be willing to go as doctor to one of the other atolls, if only we would agree to remain on Fakaofo. It seemed that no one had heard a thing that we had been saying. I had no doubt that, after our departure, they would drag Zona back out of retirement. With tongue in cheek, I suggested that he wrote his own contract this time, and set his own price. He thought this was a fabulous idea, but, as we had taken a few slurps out of his bottle by this time, I doubted whether anything would come of it. It had been raining when Dr. Zona had arrived, but, by the time he finally staggered off to his own *fale*, it was absolutely beating down, with an impressive accompaniment of thunder and lightning. This had not prevented someone from delivering a fresh baby tuna, which I found at our door.

The men from the T.P.S. visited us again, (sounds like the Terrible Person's Syndrome,) this time to ask us about a communication we had apparently received from Dr. Liutta. It was ridiculous. Any communication would have come via the official radio, to which they, and not I, had access. They would have had to forward it on to me. Perhaps there had been a letter for me, and they had just forgotten to send it across the lagoon. Or maybe it got lost in the post! Either way, I had not received it and would not have shown it to them if I had. Anyway, they said they wanted everything put down in writing. They would return for it the following morning. As far as Sue and I were concerned there would be no more writing. There would be no more of anything. The boat would be leaving in a few days – and we would be on it.

Sure enough, the following morning we saw the two of them approaching, this time with Mr. Balani waving a letter. He insisted that we had seen it previously. He was wrong. Had we seen it previously, we would have left the atoll on the last boat, and not be here waiting for the next one. Balani only read out portions of the letter and would not let me see it. Therefore I have no idea whether what he read was true, or even if it really had come from Dr. Liutta.

After about an hour and a half of meaningless verbiage, it was clear that their only concern was to get Sue and me out of the hospital. However, as two of our patients were unstable diabetics, we would be allowed to stay, as long as we kept out of the way of Tocina and Gimaima, who would be returning from suspension the following day.

Before taking their leave, they both thanked us profusely. We had got used to everyone thanking us repeatedly for what we had done and tried to do for the hospital. They said that they were taking our advice with regard to certain of our recommendations, and that the two nurses involved in all the troubles would be sent off for retraining. (I suspected that this was a blatant untruth.) We were fed up with all the mendacity and intrigue, but as we sat relaxing later that evening we had to face the possibility that this incompetence was endemic to the South Pacific area. We were listening to the National Radio of Samoa, when the announcer declared, "I have looked everywhere, but I cannot find the tape from the B.B.C., so there will be another hour of recorded music until closedown at 10.00 p.m."

We had yet another visit from Dr. Zona. It was clear that he was desperate for us to stay. He wanted to set up a meeting with Dr. Liutta, who, as well as being Director of Medical Services, was, of course, Zona's brother. It was Dr. Liutta who had requested Sue 'not to rock the boat'. He also told us that the nurses had been holding a meeting – I don't think it was at his instigation. I failed to see what they could achieve. Not only were they young, but they were also female. Together that meant that they could exert no influence over affairs on the atoll.

We had been awakened at 4.00 a.m., because Margareta's mother, who had slept through most of the previous day, was complaining that she could not sleep and had not slept for two nights. Margarita was desperate with worry. I decided that we should try some Valium to calm her mother. This would in turn give Margarita some peace of mind.

Another baby was delivered that morning. The mother did not understand when Sue complimented her on her beautiful baby, but with Leki's help was able to tell her that the baby was *'matagofie'*. She was so proud.

When I went outside, I found that someone had left out the electric pump. It was the rainy season and it had rained all night. It is hopeless to try to keep anything in good condition. I went back to bed. I was still not fully recovered from my bronchitis and the staff could cope without me, soon they would have to!

That evening we had a little feast – pickled fish and pickled onions. We only needed a bottle of Zona's home-brew to make it a completely 'pickled' evening. Instead we had to make do with some coconut juice.

The following day was 9th February. According to our original schedule we should by now have been on our way to Apia, but we were still awaiting the arrival of the boat. On the positive side, our patients were all showing signs of improvement. The blood sugars were all within acceptable limits; the baby was healthy; his mother was well and comfortable; and our little ten-year-old with the pneumonia was satisfactory. Even her tummy aches were settling down. I still couldn't make much sense of the case. Her parents had brought her in, not because of pneumonia, although she was clearly infected, but because of the abdominal pains. We were told that the child had had mumps ten days previously and that this had left her with stomach pains. It could well have been just a reaction to the mumps, but nothing was ever certain, especially in a society where it was more important to say what the listener wished to hear than to adhere too rigidly to the truth. I remained uneasy about the diagnosis.

One thing was clear; despite all the trouble with Balani, the E.O. and the two Staff Nurses, the patients still wished to be attended by me, rather than by any of the nursing staff. I found this very comforting.

We found it hard to suppress our impatience. The boat was due, but we did not know quite when it would arrive. It could be days or it could be weeks; we still had not got used to the concept of Tokelauan time. Fortunately all the diabetic patients were responding well to treatment, so we could try to relax and enjoy our remaining time on the atoll.

The local people continued to treat us as honoured guests and were very generous. That evening it was another bonito. After our experience on Tokelau, we would be able to write a book on 'Three hundred ways to serve fish', although we suspected that we would not wish to see another fish by the time we arrived back in England, not for a while anyway. When Sue returned from the main island, she had six bottles of beer, given her by the woman who ran our single little shop.

Later in the afternoon we set off for our usual walk around the island, but only got as far as the wood carver. Conversation was difficult, as he only spoke Tokelauan and our interpreter did not know how to translate the word 'skilful'. We eventually left to continue our walk and soon we met up with the Pastor's wife. She burst into tears. We had not realised that the diabetic with the badly ulcerated leg was her mother. She told us that "God in his grace had kept us on the atoll for these extra few days" especially for her mother. What could one say?

The following day we again walked across the island; this time to beg for a few litres of pure, clean water from the family who always seemed to have a supply of this precious commodity. The water from our tap appeared even more disgusting than usual and we just could not face the prospect of drinking it, even after boiling. However, when we arrived there at lunchtime, we found the whole family sound asleep. It didn't seem right to wake them up, so we left the canister on the doorstep and just continued our walk. They would not be surprised; they thought we were mad anyway. No one else would go walking in the heat of the day. I couldn't help it; I just loved the sun and the heat. Sue's usual high spirits had evaporated. She was feeling very despondent and told me that she would willingly have paid £1,000 to be able to get off the atoll at that moment. She could not stop herself continually mulling over the promises, which had been made and then so blatantly broken. I had not really expected anything, but Sue had believed them. I accepted that I was being used, but Sue felt betrayed

At about 10 o'clock that evening, Leki came around with a video cassette and asked if she and the other nurses could watch it on the player we had in the surgery. Some generous overseas donor had obviously sent this piece of brand new equipment, presumably as a teaching aid. Unfortunately no training videos had been included and, as there was no TV reception on the atoll, the machine had just stood there, looking impressive. Fortunately Gred had not yet painted over it!

It was a good film, 'The Search for Red October'; great, but just one thing wrong. The end of the tape was faulty. We did not manage to see the end of the film until much later. We mentioned it to Steve when we were back in Samoa and he just burst out laughing. It seems that it was he who had recorded the video and given it to John, who had taken it back to Tokelau. John did not have a video player, so he had passed it on to Leki. Much later we purchased a video player for John while we were on holiday in New Zealand. We bought it in the Duty Free and took it back to Samoa as part of our baggage. We spent a lovely evening drinking Steve's beer and watching the whole film again.

I couldn't say that the delay in the boat's arrival had been catastrophic, but it had certainly distressed both of us. Sue even began to get serious about the idea of hiring John's boat to sail us back to Samoa. However, the idea wouldn't work; John would have had to get the authorities in New Zealand to agree to it.

The delay of the boat had caused most of the people of the atoll to run out of flour, toilet paper, and many other essentials. We hid our meagre supply of toilet paper, or it would have vanished overnight. It was amazing that there still seemed adequate stocks of beer and cigarettes.

An Outbreak of Female Emancipation!

Life is full of surprises! The following day we were amazed to receive a delegation of ladies representing the womenfolk of Fakaofo, our atoll. Such a thing had never been seen, nor heard of, before. Apparently they had received the permission of the Elders to come and see us. I had answered a knock at the door and, when I opened it, there kneeling on the veranda was the group of women, with Dr. Zona standing to one side. They held their hands together in supplication. I beckoned to Sue. I was too overcome to say anything. Sue bade them welcome and invited them into the house. Zona indicated that he was to act as their interpreter. The ladies refused to stand up; they came in on their knees and remained kneeling all the time they were with us.

Zona explained that they had the blessing of the Elders, and now, before they spoke, could they please say a prayer? The prayer went on and on, with Zona doing his best to translate, although there was little need for translation. Their body language said everything. By this time Zona himself was in trouble. His own emotions were getting the better of him. Thank heavens,

Sue realised the situation, and she hurried off to bring him a fan. It is the custom in the South Pacific for a man to cover his face so as to hide any strong emotion. A fan is usually used for this purpose. A man must never betray his emotions in public. By now, the entire delegation was in tears. Sue had managed to get some of the older women off their knees and sitting very warily on the settee. How could we answer their pleas? It always came back to the same thing. They wanted us to stay. They insisted that the two nurses, who had caused all the problems, would be sent off for retraining, and the hospital would be handed back to us, as the only medically trained people on the atoll. They implored us to forget the insults and to withdraw our requests for an apology. Sue and I would be left to get on with the running of the hospital and with the health and well-being of the people of the atoll, without interference. It sounded appealing, but I did not see how such a prospect could possibly be acceptable to those officials who had inflated the issue to the present level. However, the delegation went off apparently satisfied with themselves, and with hugs and kisses all round. Sue had been greatly affected by the delegation, so much so that, in the end, she had promised that we would return to Fakaofo after our holiday, if everything were confirmed as they had said. I couldn't see how they would be able to achieve it.

We settled back down, to try to work as normally as possible. We had had an unusual admission to the hospital, a little girl, who had been weeping for several days and was said to have abdominal pains. When I examined her, I found all the abdominal sounds normal, with no indication of any intestinal catastrophe. I was assured that she had suffered no physical injury to explain her distress. Her parents urged me to operate, but operate on what? I refused their urgings and decided to put the little girl under observation.

Early the next morning, before the family arrived, I examined her again. This time I elicited pain over her left hip. The family insisted that the child had not been out of their sight, so could not have sustained an injury, but I was convinced that something was going on in that hip; the child was by this time running a temperature and the hip felt hot. Could it be a tubercular condition? Or might it have been a fracture? I was certain that it was not something in the abdomen, as the family kept insisting. I decided to treat it as though it was an infection and to fix the movement of the hip. The child seemed to respond to this, though every time the family moved her, we heard screams. It just had to be either a fracture, or an infection. We kept her as comfortable as we could; she started eating again – and the boat was imminent.

The two suspended nurses had not yet started back at work and, while they were away, the remaining nursing staff had become more outspoken. They demanded to be allowed to speak to Dr. Liutta, when he arrived on the next boat. They had heard that, when speaking to him, Mr. Balani had claimed to have questioned the hospital staff about what had been happening and about relationships with the suspended nurses. It was not true. He had not spoken to them and they felt very aggrieved. It was the second time that Mr. Balani had lied. The first time had been when he had claimed to have shown us Dr. Liutta's letter. He must have known that we had never seen it. One way and other, we had stirred up a hornets' nest. Never before had the women been allowed to voice an opinion.

Yet a further delegation arrived, for an 'audience' with Sue. It was the same entreaty, "Please do not leave us. We need you; we want you to stay." We found these genuine petitions very difficult to reconcile with all the lies and the back-stabbing which had occurred over the previous few weeks. I felt that Dr. Liutta would have a very hard time trying to figure it all out.

The house was beginning to resemble a place of pilgrimage. The next visitor was

Mrs. Fahrley. She was the wife of the schoolteacher, Mr. Fahrley, and, of more immediate interest to us, was the newly appointed health visitor, who would be taking over when Margareta returned to Atafu. She and her husband were among the few highly educated people on the atoll. She was also the secretary to the Women's Committee, not that that meant much, in view of the total lack of clout of any women's group on the atoll. However, she said that she thought things had now changed and would never be the same again, regardless of what happened to Sue and me. It was the first time that women's voices had been raised; what was more, she felt sure they would be heard. It was a massive step forward for the women of Tokelau. When Sue related the conversation to me, it brought to mind the ancient Greeks. In Aristophanes' classical play, Lysistrata, the women withheld their sexual favours from their husbands, forcing them to end the long war between Athens and Sparta. The woman of Fakaofo had not gone to these extremes, but it was at least a first step.

The following day, we received an invitation from the teachers of the school, but to what we were invited, we had no idea. The invitation was written in Tokelauan. We were just wondering whom we should ask to translate it for us, when the headmaster himself arrived, huffing and puffing. The invitation was a mistake; we should have received an English version. It turned out, there was to be a party and we were urged to attend.

We were pleased that we did. It was a good party. The food was good, although a trifle late arriving, and the drink was wonderful, particularly one made from two-day-old fermented coconut tree sap; it was like nectar. It reminded me of a visit to Germany at the time of the grape harvest. There we paid two pounds for two glasses of freshly-squeezed grape juice. It didn't taste as good as our two-day fermented coconut. The two-day fermentation was crucial. It produced a good, full-bodied taste. Three-day grog may have been stronger, but it was too rough for my taste.

After a very quite period in the hospital, suddenly the wards were full again. Among the new patients was an eight-year-old girl, who had fallen about 20 feet from a coconut tree, when an insect had flown into her eye. Unfortunately there was an obvious fracture; with no X-ray or anaesthetic available I had to see what I could do for her. Dr. Zona came to see if he could help. I then remembered the ampoules of dental anaesthetic in the back of the cupboard, I diluted one of these down with some normal saline, and putting the girl on to our so called operating couch, injected the fracture sight with enough local to make her pain free. Then with Dr. Zona holding on to her, I pulled her arm straight, and with the help of two flat bits of wood the nurse proceeded to bandage her arm. The child eventually sat up feeling a little wobbly but none the worst for ware. But I would have to keep my eye on her and her makeshift splint. She was another patient that would have to go to Samoa to have it checked by an X-ray. But I was sure that all would be well.

The other little girl was not doing so well and her temperature was fluctuating wildly. Still no one would admit to her having sustained any injury, but her hip just did not feel right. Worryingly her weight was going down. To be on the safe side, I decided to start her on a course of anti-tuberculosis treatment. Life would have been much easier if we had had a laboratory, or an X-ray machine, but, of course, we had none of these. Even the inter-island catamaran was not available for an emergency transfer to Samoa. We had to rely on our own resources; there was no back-up.

During this period we were badly infested with mosquitoes. Sue and I found their buzzing and biting almost intolerable, but none of the patients seemed to notice; the reason, there was an important rugby game about to start. It was the Pacific seven-a-side tournament and it was being broadcast on the radio. The Samoan team were Pacific Champions and they were hosting a game against one of the other South Pacific islands. As usual the introductions began at least half an hour before the game was due to begin. The first was a speech in English by a Samoan government minister. It was clear that he himself did not understand a word of English and had no idea what he was saying. Someone had obviously written the speech for him. However, as few of his audience understood English either, it probably did not matter one iota that it was incomprehensible gibberish. The main thing was that it took up the allotted time. It was followed by a long prayer, asking for blessings on all and sundry, but especially for the health of the minister, and of his family, and of his relatives, and of his friends. The proceedings were continuously interrupted with cries from the relatives, hangers-on, business colleagues and supporters, of "*malo malo*". Like many Samoan phrases, this can have many meanings, but we were assured that on this occasion it meant "Well done." We could not guess whether this was a reference to the minister's last explanation to the newspapers as to why the state airline had gone bankrupt, or to another on the beneficial effect of the proposed introduction of VAT on the health and well-being of the people of Samoa. *Malo malo* was the cry and the people joined in happily. The prayer would probably have continued long into the night, had it not been for the rugby match. There was just time for a final "Thanks be to God; Amen" and it was time for the kick-off. The prayer obviously had the desired effect, either through the power of the Almighty, or by lulling the visiting team into a coma. Whichever it was, they were soundly trounced by Samoa. There was much home-brew sunk on the atoll that night, even in the hospital.

Amazingly, by the following morning, the little girl's temperature had dropped dramatically and she had started eating again. It was an encouraging sign.

The rumour mill had been busy again. Apparently the Women's Committee had issued a demand to Dr. Liutta that Tocina and Gimaima had to be sent off the atoll. What a hope! Another rumour probably had more substance. This was to the effect that the Elders wished to close down Neta's radio receiver. They continued to fret at the fact that she always got information before they did. It was inevitable, as John had high quality radio equipment on board his boat. He also had many friends both in Samoa and on Tokelau. John was always the first to receive any titbits of information and he simply passed them on to Neta. Now the Elders wanted to put a stop to it. I didn't see how they could possibly do so. It would be a limitation on freedom of speech; a violation of her human rights...... Oh, I had forgotten; we were on Tokelau: such considerations did not apply. Still, I could not prevent myself from voicing my opinion. I told the *Faipule* that only the Minister of Posts and Telegraphs in New Zealand would be able to authorise such action and, even then, there would have to be a convincing argument that Neta's possession of a radio receiver breached national security. It was obvious from Melli's expression that I was just whistling in the wind. Just as in the story from Samoa, the Elders of Fakaofo did not welcome interference from outside. They were a law unto themselves. I left them to it. Anyway, if what they were transmitting was so damned confidential, why did they not filter it through a scrambler unit? They were cheap enough. I had even used one back in Yorkshire, in order to speak to Sue at home while doing house calls.

Melli parried my criticism with an invitation. The Elders wished us to attend a party. It would be another gesture of appreciation for all we had done and urging us, once again, to return to Tokelau after our holiday. I expressed our thanks for the invitation and our pleasure at their kind thoughts towards us. However, I explained that it was only Dr. Liutta, as Medical Director, who could give us the assurances we needed, and I would give the Elders our final decision after we had spoken to him.

Even our neighbouring wood carver appeared to be in on the conspiracy. He informed me that the carvings would be ready for me on my return from holiday. Talk about blackmail! It would have taken a little more than that inducement to get us to come back.

The little girl's temperature was going up and down, but at least she was eating well. However, she would not let me touch her hip. Either there must be pus in it, or, despite what her parents were saying, it must be fractured. I was determined to get her to Samoa for an X-ray, even though the *Faipule* had told me that the atoll could not afford the charges which would be levied by the hospital in Apia. The boat was on its way and I would get her on it.

Later that evening, I was approached by another of the Elders, the husband of one of our recent admissions to the hospital. He said that he wished to read the E.O.'s letter. I was surprised; I thought that its contents were now common knowledge, but apparently not. After reading it, he left in an absolute fury. I could only conclude that the E.O. and his friends were still trying to pervert the truth concerning the contents of the letter.

It was time for one last round of the wards before bed. The little girl was resting peacefully and her temperature was back to normal.

The following morning, I did the usual clinic and then went back to bed and slept for the rest of the morning. Although I had recovered from my bronchitis, I was still not feeling fully fit and the rest did me good.

When I awoke, it was pouring with rain. It was the middle of the rainy season. The rain was warm and refreshing, so I splashed through it across to the hospital. While rummaging about in some cupboards, I found a few ampoules of Heavy Nupercain. Unfortunately they were over five years out of date – and the long spinal needles were broken. It was all so depressing.

There seems to be a dispute going on between the Elders in connection with the new (or nearly new) boat which has been acquired. It appears that it is actually on hire to the atolls, at vast cost and the Elders of the three atolls wish to control its use – in particular, they wish to ensure that they will be able to use it for their own private and pleasurable purposes. It infuriated me that there was money for such luxuries, but yet they apparently could not afford the cost of a hospital bed in Apia. I was determined that my young patient would go to Apia come what may, even if it meant that I had to carry her aboard the boat myself.

Another function was planned for the following day and we were invited. The Elders had declared a *Fono*, which meant meeting, and included a six day feast. The native word for it was *Fufui* – to bake a pig. How they could organise a feast on an island which had run out of flour, rice and many other commodities – not to mention toilet paper – I could not imagine. I sometimes had to despair at their priorities. I wondered if they deserved to survive in the modern world. For anyone who wished to spend his life doing nothing at all, then this was the place to do it. Nothing mattered on Tokelau.

I could not get the young girl out of my mind. I questioned her parents again, but they continued to insist that she had been running about after her fall two weeks earlier.

Certainly the child was suffering from pneumonia when she had been brought in to us. But what else and why? I wrote out the child's history, as given to me by the parents, which I would pass on to the hospital in Apia. However, I added that, although I had described the background as it had been given to me, I was not convinced of the veracity of it. I believed that the left hip was the real trouble and that it could be a fracture or a dislocation, which explained my reason for not attempting to manipulate it but only to immobilise it. The parents were really very appreciative of all that we had tried to do. They had been so certain that they had only brought their child into the hospital to die.

Despite our misgivings, we decided to attend the function the following afternoon. We asked our boat driver to stand by to take us to the other island. He forgot! We had to 'thumb a lift' from our neighbour. We didn't actually see our driver until it was time to come back across the lagoon after the meeting.

We were again the guests of honour at the meeting. There were speeches and presentations from everyone, including from the Women's Committee. We received gifts from nearly every family on the atoll. All were hand-made and each was presented to us by the family, which had made it. Some were sleeping mats (On Tokelau, no one could imagine sleeping on anything other than a sleeping mat.) and some of them were so big that it took the whole family to lift them. Some had designs, which were so intricate that the weaving of them must have taken weeks. I anticipated some difficulty in getting the mats back to Samoa. How on earth were we going to get them back to England?

Sue was going through her usual ritual of cleaning up, leaving everything in pristine condition for the next resident. We had decimated the population of pests during our stay, so at least it should be much more pleasant to live in. We were particularly sensitive. We did not like the insects and other wildlife, whereas the natives accepted the cockroaches as equal inhabitants.

Dr. Zona called in for a few farewell drinks; he had been off to talk with, as he said, *peoples*. He was really up-tight and very hurt. He spoke about Tocina. Although she was his relative, he viewed her with great bitterness. He could never forget the incident where, exerting her authority, she had stopped him operating on a patient, who had subsequently died. I observed that there could only be one captain on a ship, and it required someone who was competent, reliable or trustworthy. I did not need to spell out that, in my view, Tocina fulfilled none of the requirements.

Sue continued to take a leading part in the running of the hospital and, while I sat talking with Dr. Zona, she did the evening round of the wards. Everything was in order and all the patients were comfortable. When she returned, we pushed Zona off to his bed and took ourselves off to ours.

The Arrival of the Boat – And Farewell to Tokelau!

In the morning I noticed two radiograms on the table in the hospital. They were addressed to the 'M.O. and Staff Nurse in charge'. That made the situation very clear to me. It was Monday morning and I was being given the 'Zona treatment'. Sure enough, later in the morning, Tocina turned up for work. She was back at full blast, dishing out pills to all and sundry, regardless of the ailment and with nothing being recorded. All Sue's careful work was being destroyed in a single morning. I went back to the house in disgust, to be followed shortly after by Leki. The poor girl was in tears. It was not long before patients began to bypass the hospital and come directly to our residence asking for help. We found it very difficult to cope with. Everything was falling to pieces under our noses.

We learned that the boat was due to arrive that afternoon. It would disembark some of the passengers and would then carry on to the two other atolls, before returning to Fakaofo for a general *fono* and to pick up passengers for Apia. Margareta's mother had already gone across to the main island, ready to board the boat for the trip to Atafu. Her diabetes had been stabilised and she was greatly improved. However, I had learned that Atafu held virtually no medical supplies, so the longer-term prognosis for the patient was not very good.

Dr. Zona came to see us, beaming like a Cheshire cat. He had had a meeting with his brother, Dr. Liutta, who had arrived on the boat. Zona had explained everything to him and he told us that he believed that we had been given a massive vote of confidence, together with a large bottle of vodka. He also brought us a letter from the Medical Director, couched in the friendliest of terms. Dr. Zona was positively bubbling over, but Sue was much more dubious about it all.

Some packages were delivered from the boat. I was hopeful that it was the textbooks for the nurses, which I had requested from Apia. In the absence of a doctor, they would at least be able to look up the symptoms and gain some idea. When we had arrived, there had not been a single medical textbook on the atoll. The packages did not contained books, just another set, or rather four sets, of chest spreaders. Absolutely brilliant! On this tiny atoll, in the middle of the South Pacific, with no doctor, no serviceable operating theatre and no anaesthetics, the powers-that-be had decided that the most urgent need was for chest spreaders.

By the Friday of that week, 18th February 1994, the boat was back again from Atafu. It would leave for Apia on the following Monday. Our little girl with the funny hip was running a temperature again, but now she would let me move her hip a little without screaming and she was also beginning to put a little flesh back on. There seemed to be problem getting her a berth on the boat. Sue went off to sort that out. If it really came to it, we were prepared to pay for her passage ourselves.

When Sue returned, she had with her a beautifully carved turtle, a gift from the parents of little Max. She also brought a fistful of mail. One of the letters was from the Medical Director. It had apparently been sent to us by radio telephone in January. It was so insulting that, had we received it at that time, we would have left Tokelau on the earlier boat, regardless of any other considerations. What on earth could the director have been thinking about? Of course, at the back of our minds, we knew well enough. Tocina had been sending off radio messages from the transmitter on the other island.

We had our own little party on the Saturday night. John and Neta arrived, together with Dr. Zona, and they brought a large quantity of beer from the boat. It was a good night.

On the Sunday morning I carried out a suction clearance on one of the children who had arrived on the boat, clearing out a very dirty and infected ear. Meanwhile Dr. Zona went to pick up the new delivery of drugs for the hospital.

We were being inundated with visitors, well-wishers and people bringing yet more gifts. The big fellow, the husband of the diabetic patient who had nearly died, brought in his gift. He was one of the Elders and also one of the atoll's great fishermen. He brought me a hand-made shark hook; it was magnificent, made of wood and coconut fibre. It really was something to see. We also received a number of hand-carved native boats and Sue suddenly acquired a large number of hats, all beautifully made. How we would get it all back to Samoa, let alone back to England, was a mystery.

On that, our final evening, a party was held in the hospital in our honour. I can't really say that we were in party mood, but we could not refuse. What a banquet! There were more crabs and many other delicacies. The people must have been cooking for days. The food was fantastic. We wondered how they had managed to keep it all so secret. After about an hour, we were approached, first by Gimaima and then by Tocina. In front of everyone they abased themselves begged our forgiveness. They said that they had done wrong. Gimaima said that her husband, the E.O. and a lay preacher, had relieved himself of all preaching duties, as he also knew that he had done wrong. Tocina followed with her catalogue of failings. What else could we do but graciously forgive them. We certainly would never forget. And of course, now that they had apologised, we would have to come back. What con merchants they were!

Zona closed off the evening with prayers, but by this time he was well and truly under the influence and he got himself a wee bit mixed up. He quoted something from Deuteronomy, but we didn't really make much sense of it; and so we retired to bed, tired and somewhat inebriated. It was already 1:30 a.m. Final thought – "Is this the beginning of the end or the end of another beginning?"

Our journey to the boat was very slow and meandering. Nearly the whole atoll turned out to see us off, and we had to go and see those who were not able to come down to the water's edge. It was a very emotional farewell. We said goodbye to the parents of Max Marlo and Mini Sue. They were still asking us to return. If only things had been different. Sue and I knew in our heart of hearts that there would be no coming back. We could not believe a single word of their promises: but we had done our best and we had fallen in love with them – the people of Tokelau.

Back to Samoa

The boat was an eye-opener. It was magnificent – particularly to Sue and me, who had become used to the inadequacy of facilities on Tokelau. As soon as we were aboard, we were met by the captain, who in turn introduced us to the owners and the rest of the crew. Whereas the captain was originally from England, the crew were mainly German mariners.

We were invited to cocktails and, after drinking toasts to all and sundry, we were shown to our cabin, or rather to our suite. The boat's owners had kindly offered us what turned out to be literally the Royal Suite.

The boat was one of three identical vessels, built for the Australian Coastguard Service, to service lighthouses and other coastal installations. During a royal tour of Australia, the Queen had sailed on this particular boat, the Cape Don, and we were now installed in what had been her cabin.

Although the Cape Don was in private ownership, it might have been very different. It seems that, after the sad demise of the previous boat, the Queen Salamasina, the Tokelauans were given the opportunity to purchase the Cape Don for £100,000. The Elders decided that this was too much, so it was sold instead to the businessmen whom we had just met. They chartered it back to Tokelau, for the trip from Samoa to the Atolls, at a cost of £10,000 per voyage. At about eight trips each year, it didn't take much to work out who had made the best deal!

After an emotionally tiring day, we retired to bed in the Royal Suite, determined not to dwell on the recent frustrations, but to look forward to the next part of our adventure, to life in Western Samoa.

The following day, en route to Samoa, Sue found a bar of chocolate in the freezer. She had not seen chocolate for over six months. It was just too much of a temptation. Unfortunately frozen chocolate is as hard as iron, and when it came to the question of which would give way first, the chocolate or Sue's teeth, it was no contest. And so it was that Sue arrived in Samoa with one broken tooth.

We had left Fakaofo at about 5.00 p.m. on Monday 21st February and had expected to dock at Apia around 9.00 p.m. the following day. We were therefore surprised when we carried on to a smaller port further up the coast. This was probably due to the high charges for docking facilities at Apia. We had been told that a car would be waiting for us, but there was no car to be seen. After some hours and much telephoning, a car did eventually turn up. Maybe life on Samoa would not be so different to Tokelau after all!

We piled our luggage into the back of the car, no easy task, considering the vast array of lovingly made gifts from Fakaofo, and set off for Steve's house, where we were to stay until our flight left four days later. Our trip to New Zealand had been postponed, but, thanks to Steve, we were booked to fly from Apia to Auckland on 26th February.

Steve and Ava welcomed us with open arms, and the first question, "Tell us all about it." Sue was impatient to catch up on all the news – and most of all, to find out about the wedding. It seems that Steve had been thwarted in his wish for a quiet wedding and Ava had prevailed. It had been a traditional Samoan ceremony, with Ava in white, and with Taimani as her bridesmaid. Steve had dressed in a white shirt and white lava-lava, with a traditional headband of green foliage. The wedding service had been conducted by Ava's brother-in-law, a church minister in Samoa. Steve and Ava had danced the afternoon away, but had then left for their honeymoon on his motorcycle, with tin cans tied to the back, making a fearful noise as they rode off into the setting sun. We were pleased to note that Steve had not completely abandoned his principles!

After we had exhausted the subject of the wedding, Steve was anxious to hear how we had fared on Fakaofo. He was not surprised by any of it. He had also had his arguments with the same Medical Director. What was surprising to us was how much of our story he already knew. He must also have been able to tap into John and Neta's well of news and rumour.

We had so much to catch up on, but eventually we tore ourselves away, as we needed to go into Apia to sort out the situation concerning the refrigerator. We explained to the company supplying it, that it would be of little use on Fakaofo until they had a stable power supply. To our surprise, they understood the situation perfectly and assured us that it was no problem at all. The money was refunded and we had it sent back to the charity which had donated it.

Having sorted this out to our satisfaction, we went off to see Dr. Liutta, the Medical Director for Tokelau. What a waste of an afternoon! Firstly he was rather upset that we had cancelled the refrigerator, even though he could not guarantee the power supply to run it. This seemed to be typical of the general mind-set of those running Tokelau – accumulate as much equipment as possible, regardless of whether it was of any practical use.

Then, while we had already decided that our time in Tokelau was over, Dr. Liutta was clearly determined that I should go back. He suggested that, after our holiday, I should be prepared to go to one of the other atolls to continue the work I had done on Fakaofo. He finished by suggesting that, while in New Zealand, I should write a paper on the benefits of one centralised hospital serving the three atolls of Tokelau, and how such an outcome could be attained. I found it very significant that Sue did not feature in his plans. He may live on Samoa, but his attitude to women was no different to that which still pertained on Tokelau.

I responded that I had read his last communication to me very carefully and felt that his advice was incorrect. Furthermore I considered his conclusions, which amounted to a set of demands, to be very foolish. To my astonishment he went into a long and involved explanation, saying that he regretted some of the things he had written.

We left Dr. Liutta on the understanding that, while on holiday, I would consider all he had said. In reality our minds were already made up. There was no way that I was going to work for the Tokelauan authorities again, and certainly not for Dr. Liutta.

On leaving Dr. Liutta's office, we made our way to the National Hospital, where we enquired about the progress of our young patient. As I had suspected, X-rays had confirmed a dislocation of the hip. Once it was clear that there was no fracture, it was a relatively simple procedure to manipulate the joint back into position. By the time we arrived, she was already well on the way to a full recovery and was smiling happily and looking much better than when we had last seen her.

Having dealt with the business side of things, it was time to sort out Sue's broken tooth. Through Steve, we had already met one of the doctors working in Apia. Jacky was from New Zealand and probably one of the best of the doctors on Samoa. She suggested that Sue wait until we reached New Zealand, where her brother was a dental consultant in Christchurch. It would all be set up for Sue. He would see her himself. No problem! And so it turned out. No problem!

We had been back in Samoa a few days. It was already approaching the end of February. Where on earth did the time go?

The previous night we had been out to Aggie Gray's for a meal. Aggie's was a place where Sue and I would have loved to have stayed, even just for one night. It had the reputation as the best hotel on the island and was very popular with the Americans (because of James Mitchener's book, I supposed) and with the Germans, who, with the strength of the Deutschmark at that time, were major world travellers. But Sue had hold of the purse strings and she said "No." It would have cost well over £100 sterling per night and Sue decided that that exceeded our budget. In any case, the food was not *that* good. However, we did go there for several meals and for drinks. We also used Aggie's as a pick-up point. They had a bus, which took guests to the airport, and we could join that without actually having to stay at the hotel.

The Japanese were investing more and more in Samoa. Shortly before our visit they had bought the Tusitalia hotel, the largest hotel in Apia after Aggie's. They were still busy refurbishing it and hiring new staff. They would give Aggie's a run for their money, as the saying goes.

Anyway, back to the story; leaving the restaurant, we had taken a taxi. We noticed that the driver was already slightly intoxicated when we got into his cab and he kept topping himself up from a bottle at his side, until we arrived at our destination. Then he asked us for twenty five dollars for a five dollar fare. After some argument, he drove off without any payment at all. He was definitely drunk!

A Visit to New Zealand and Tonga

Finally it was time to depart for our long-awaited holiday trip to New Zealand. Our doctor friend, Jacky, picked us up at 2.00 a.m. on Saturday 26th February 1994 and drove us down to Aggie's, where we caught the bus to the airport. I had helped Jacky out by seeing a few of her patients and she was happy to return the favour.

During the flight to Auckland, we crossed the International Date Line once again. Samoa is just to the east of the I.D.L. and New Zealand just to its west. Therefore in flying from Apia to Auckland, we lost a day. We left Samoa at about 5.00 a.m. on 26th and, after a six hour flight, arrived in New Zealand at around mid-day on 27th February. It was all very confusing. My wristwatch had already given up. For the length of our stay in New Zealand, I had to accept that the date function was set to Samoan time, rather than to that of the real world.

This book is not intended as a travelogue of New Zealand, so I will gloss over that part of our trip. Suffice it to say that we had a splendid holiday. Sue had her tooth repaired and the dentist and his family entertained us right royally. After touring the various wine districts, we travelled over the spine of the Southern Alps in South Island to meet up with Julian Ashburner, a doctor from our own area of Yorkshire. He had emigrated to a small town near Graymouth on the west coast. We spent a wonderful few days with him and his friends, so much so that we even toyed with the idea of buying the small bungalow next to his property. It was on offer at a very reasonable price. New Zealand and its people were wonderful. The country reminded me of Britain as it had been before the last war.

We left New Zealand after about three weeks, but, instead of flying directly back to Samoa, we stopped off for a week in Tonga. Sue was most disappointed. Queen Salote's visit to London for the Coronation in 1953 had fired her imagination and the wish to visit the islands had stayed with her for all those years. That was our main reason for visiting Tonga. It is enough to say that we both wish we hadn't. It was drab and unkempt. The hotels were all run down and the entire island looked in need of refurbishment. From what little we saw, we concluded that Captain Cook had been deceived when he had named them the 'The Friendly Isles' and the islanders certainly did not appear friendly or helpful to tourists. As for the royal family, it seemed that the king spent the all country's meagre wealth on building houses for himself and his relatives.

However, one thing did come out of our visit. The receptionist at our hotel gave me an introduction to Dr. Afeaki, the Secretary of the Tongan Medical Association. He offered me work on Tonga's most beautiful island, starting immediately. He said that the hardest work would be teaching and supervising. It sounded very attractive, but we had found out, to our cost, that everything in the South Pacific had a catch to it. Still, it was good to have the feeling that we had something to fall back on, if we were to need it. Dr. Afeaki asked me to provide my C.V., as soon as was practical. As the hospital in Apia had at least two copies in their files, that would present no problem.

Looking for Work
(or Wheels within Wheels)

Upon our return to Apia on 28th March, I went straight to the hospital. They spent all day trying to find my C.V., but with no success. I was totally fed up. No one seemed to know where anything was. Finally Sue and I went off to the Post Office, from where we telephoned one of our daughters back home in Yorkshire. She agreed to photo-copy all my degrees, diplomas, etc. and fax them to me in Apia.

A couple of days later, on 30th March, Steve took us out to lunch. We were not alone. He had also invited another English girl to join us. She was being sponsored by S.P.R.E.P. (South Pacific Regional Educational Programme) to study the marine mollusc population. We were never sure of the purpose of her investigation. She had been having trouble filling her diving tanks and Steve was trying to obtain a compressor for her. When she eventually succeeded in getting the tanks filled, it was with the assistance of the local brewery – in view of this last statement, I should emphasise that it was oxygen and not beer that they put into the tanks. Steve insisted that she should test them using her own pressure gauges – and that proved to be wise advice, for she found that they were only half full. Perhaps this explained why the oxygen cylinders sent to Tokelau had also been only half-full. Could it be that they had been provided by the same brewery?

The following day was Good Friday and we had been invited to meet up with the Hash Harriers again. We would have a long weekend on Savaii, the other main island of Western Samoa. It was reminiscent of our previous visit of 1990, although signs of the hurricane which had struck during the intervening period were clearly evident. We again visited the blowholes and we clambered up to a volcano. Sue and some of the others climbed down inside and even went for a swim in the crater lake. We visited waterfalls, lava flows and deserted beaches, such a contrast with the endless coral sand of Fakaofo. On the Monday morning, 4th April, we got up very early and watched the sun rise over the Pacific Ocean. The whole weekend had been magical and we returned to Apia that evening weary but exhilarated.

The Thursday of that week marked a special occasion. It was 7th April and Sue's birthday. We had hoped to take out Steve, Ava and her sister, Taimani, to celebrate. However, Steve and Ava had a previous engagement, so we just went with Taimani. We had booked a table at the Waterfront Restaurant in the centre of town. We were told that it was the best place to eat, not only in Apia, but in the whole of Western Samoa. It lived up to its reputation; we had a splendid meal and Taimani introduced us to the two ladies who ran the restaurant. One, Miss Adrianne, was a New Zealander and the other, Malu, a Samoan. After the meal we went off to a party where we stayed until very late. As Taimani was driving us home, Sue noticed a deep red glow in the sky and, being curious, Taimani turned off towards it. We soon realised that the glow came from the restaurant at which we had dined earlier in the evening and that it was ablaze. By the time we arrived there, a small crowd had gathered. Already rumours were rife. No one was in any doubt that the fire had been started deliberately and most people seemed confident that they even knew who had done it. One thing was sure; the best restaurant in town was disappearing in front of our eyes. It seemed that it had been too successful. Someone had decided that the market economy was better without too much competition.

The next few weeks were taken up with me looking for employment and Sue helping out as 'housekeeper' for Steve and Ava. I had various meetings in the hospital in Apia and, in between, treated a few patients to 'keep my hand in'. However, it was all rather frustrating. Here was a country with very limited medical resources and yet it seemed impossible to cut through the red tape of bureaucracy.

I was beginning to get a little disheartened when, towards the end of April, Steve asked if I would be prepared to see a friend of his, who was worried by a medical condition. Obviously I agreed and we arranged to meet the following day.

The next morning, Steve took us into Apia and into one of the few modern buildings in the town. We soon realised that these prestigious offices belonged to a firm of high-powered lawyers, Svensen and Company. In fact, Terry Svensen himself turned out to be the legal adviser to the Samoan Prime Minister. Terry was a large, overweight New Zealander, bursting with energy and obviously enjoying life. There was immediate empathy between us and, in the course of time, we became good friends. He was instrumental in sorting out many of our difficulties. When it came to dealing with bureaucracy and red tape, Terry was Mr. Fixit!

However, the purpose of our visit on that morning was ostensibly of a medical nature, so I enquired what the problem was. It turned out to be to be a large ulcer on his leg – which he hoped I would be able to sort out. It seemed that it had all started with a couple of little insect bites, which had rapidly turned nasty. He had been treated by the local doctors but to no avail. When he learned of it, Steve mentioned me – and that was how we came to be in Terry's office. Sue cleaned up the wound with hot water and peroxide, and I applied the powder from one of my capsules of antibiotic. We covered it with a light bandage and advised Terry that we would need to repeat the procedure several times until the wound started to heal.

Before we left, Terry invited us to his home that evening for drinks.

We had difficulty finding his house, despite the clear instructions. Just when we thought we were there, we found ourselves in the middle of what seemed to be a derelict circus, complete with big top. Terry later explained to us that he knew the owner, who was desperate to find somewhere to park his circus, at a reasonable price. Terry had generously agreed to help out.

The house was built on a large spit of land, jutting out into a small bay, with a small islet shielding it from the open sea. The house itself was as beautiful as its surroundings and its view. Terry's wife, Luanna, had been a onetime winner of the Miss World competition. Despite having raised a family, she had retained her good looks and figure, which was unusual in that part of the world. Their children were being educated in New Zealand.

The evening was a great success, with tasty refreshment and convivial conversation. Terry insisted on hearing our story, from how we came to meet Steve Brown (or perhaps more precisely, how we came to meet his hat!), through our adventures on Tokelau, right up to our current predicament. At the end, he just said, "I'll arrange for you to see the Prime Minister." He made it sound so easy, as if we had not been trying to speak to someone in authority ever since we had arrived back from Tokelau. Even the consultants at the hospital had been unable to get us an appointment with a minister.

We were at breakfast a couple of days later, when we received a call from Terry, "Best bib and tucker, down at my office, 11 o'clock!" The '11 o'clock' was fine. It was the 'best bib and tucker' that presented the problem. Steve's house stood off the beaten track, in fact, about twenty minutes walk through the fields to the nearest bus stop – and it was pouring with rain. The fields were a quagmire. We had to carry our decent clothes in a bag. By the time we arrived at the Svensen offices in the centre of Apia, we looked as if we had just come through a battlefield. We were in no state to meet the doorman, let alone the Prime Minister. Fortunately Terry's office complex was equipped with a bathroom, complete with hot and cold running water, soap and even clean towels. Thank heavens! It was wonderful how a good wash and a change of clothes could make everything seem so much better.

The Prime Minister's office was only about five minutes walk away from Terry's office. It occupied the top floor of a relatively new building that had been designed and built by the Chinese. The fascia and much of the décor had been finished in an awful yellowish plastic. The whole area looked rather run-down, as indeed did most of the people waiting to be seen. They looked as if they had come straight from the paddy fields. Terry corrected us: this was their Sunday best. They were petitioners sent by their villages as being their most articulate spokesmen. They would be asking for something or other for their villages.

Whilst Sue and I were waiting, in came one of the consultants from the hospital, a Dr. Atta. He was one of those who had genuinely tried to help us, but he himself had problems. He had apparently trodden on someone's toes. He had not been given consultancy status when every one else had been upgraded. Maybe it was just that he had qualified in New Zealand, whereas all the others had Tongan, Fijian or other 'local' degrees. Anyway I found him very helpful and competent. Terry had arranged for Dr. Atta to join us in the meeting with the Prime Minister, His Highness Malietoa Tanumafili II.

Eventually we were ushered into the Prime Minister's office. It was a very large room, one side of which obviously served as an office, and the other portion furnished as a comfortable lounge.

We were greeted most formally in English, and Dr. Atta made the introductions. The P.M. wasted no time. "What organisation do you represent?" he asked me. "None," I replied. "We have funded everything ourselves." A look of utter disbelief spread over his face. "Why?" he asked. His questions were short and to the point. I had the impression that he was a busy man, who had no time for small talk. However, after a few moments, he stopped me and said, "Come." On saying this, he got up from behind his desk and motioned Sue, me and Dr. Atta to follow him across to the lounge area. He seated himself in a large easy chair; the P.M. was a large man, and motioned Sue and me to a large settee and Dr. Atta to a separate armchair. "Now start at the beginning. How did you come here in the beginning and why?"

At the end of our story, he just turned to Dr. Atta and said. "Is he any good?"

Dr. Atta replied to the effect that my background had been checked out by his office and by the hospital and the answer to his question was, "Yes, he is good." "Hire him then," and then turning to me he said, "I want you on my home." By this he meant the other island, Savaii, and that was how it came about that we kept our promise, made four years earlier to the matron of the hospital at Palauli, that we would return to Savaii.

Before we could leave Apia and travel to the Samoa's most westerly island of Savaii, we had to resolve a few little difficulties with our visas and work permits. Our visas were for a limited period, but for most of the time we had been on Tokelau. Despite this fact, the Passport Office showed no inclination to extend the visas and claimed that we had already overstayed our allotted stay. I had no work permit and the Passport Office was claiming that I owed money for previous permits. The atmosphere was somewhat strained and, rather than get into further argument, we decided to return to Terry's office. It was a wonderful experience to watch someone pick up the telephone and just say, "Get me the Prime Minister." It was like watching a Hollywood movie – "Get me the Prime Minister!" Soon I had a letter, confirming my appointment to serve as Doctor in Charge of the hospital at Sataua and informing me that I would receive a small allowance to help with our living expenses. Then the following day we received our passports, all signed up correctly and with no charge this time, and handed over with a smile.

The Island of Savaii

On 20th May 1994 we set sail again. After the luxury of the Cape Don, it was a bit of a comedown. We could not imagine anything looking less sea-worthy. It seemed to be a remnant from the Second World War, a modified tank landing craft – and it was leaking. The bow doors were definitely not watertight, but no-one else seemed concerned, so, as the vessel did the trip twice a day, we decided that it must be reasonably safe. Well that was what we kept saying to ourselves. The thing that nearly scuppered us was not the condition of the boat, but something totally unforeseen. Just as we were about to set sail, a car came speeding down to the dockside, hooting and tooting like mad. It was our driver and, in his haste, he nearly drove off the end of the jetty. On his way back to Apia after dropping us off, he had met the hospital director coming the other way. They had forgotten to give us the keys to our new home. One thing we had learned: life was never dull in the South Pacific.

A clapped out, flat-topped vehicle met us at the small jetty at Salelologa and our belongings were quickly loaded. We were beginning to look like travelling gypsies, with our suitcases, white plastic boxes, brown paper parcels and woven baskets. I am sure that, back in the U.K., we would have been regarded with great suspicion, whereas on Savaii we were treated like royalty.

After a two hour drive we arrived at the hospital in Sataua, where we planned to live and work for the next four months. Our friendly driver had been chatting away in very presentable English. He told us that our new home had been locked up since the last doctor left, well over a year previously. He had departed in a haze of oriental drugs – and the telephone company were still trying to get their bill paid! Well at least we had the keys.

As the hospital came into sight, we could see that it was built on a larval flow, jutting out into the sea, about ten feet above sea level. It looked like a teardrop laid out in the surf. The hospital itself consisted of one large single-storied block on the right. Standing opposite were three bungalows and one ruined wreck of a bungalow. The driver cheerfully informed us that that one was the doctor's home, unfortunately destroyed by the last hurricane. We were aghast. Of what use were a set of keys, when there was no front door? "But you will nice place live in," he continued. "Girls all are cleaning it lovely."

With a rousing squawk from the horn of his clapped out vehicle, he drew up in front of the hospital, producing an eruption of women from all corners. A statuesque figure in a crisp white uniform strode forward and introduced herself as Alua. We never learned her full name, so forever afterwards she remained just Alua. She apologised for not having everything in good order. They had only been informed that morning that we were arriving and so the whole hospital staff had been busy cleaning our quarters. A glance of relief passed between us. We were to have a house after all. We were therefore rather surprised when Alua continued that the ward was ready for us. We had expected to go straight to our house to unpack and tidy up, rather than to start an immediate inspection of the hospital. Seeing our puzzled looks, she explained that, as the doctor's house had been destroyed, they had done their best to turn the maternity ward into a home for us. With that, Alua opened the door of the erstwhile maternity unit, "An electrician coming in the morning to repair cooker," she said, "tonight nurses invite all to their house, nurses' home, to eat, please."

We were left alone and at last had the chance to assess our new environment. All the hospital buildings, including the maternity unit, seemed to be built on identical concrete bases, with an entrance door in the centre of one side. This opened into a spacious hall, which would be our lounge, with smaller rooms to the right and left. On the left side was a toilet room and next to it a sluice room, which was to be our kitchen. Opposite this, and on the other side of the 'lounge', was a bedroom containing a double bed and a wardrobe. To the right of that, nearest to the entrance door, was another room with a single bed in it. The hall, which we had already worked out was to be our lounge, contained a large table. Obviously our hall/lounge was to be our hall/lounge/dining room!

In front to the table, at the opposite end of the room to the main entrance, was a large window, taking up nearly the whole of the wall area. What a view! We were looking down the larval flow as it had poured out to sea. We had an uninterrupted view of the tropical shore, the Pacific Ocean and the sky.

It looked as if we would be reasonably comfortable, provided that the hospital admitted no maternity patients!

As we looked around, we thought back to our arrival in Tokelau. Here we did at least have an electric stove, even if it did need repairing. But there were no cooking pots or utensils. Thank goodness we had brought a small travelling kettle. We turned the tap and water came out. What's more, it looked relatively clean. Unfortunately the contents of the cupboards looked very familiar, the same odious black cockroaches were in residence.

There was other livestock to keep us company too. They seemed to live on the walls and ceilings, and they were geckoes. We developed rather a love/hate relationship with them. They turned out to be rather interesting animals or, more precisely, reptiles. They would come out in the evenings and Sue and I spent many hours absorbed in watching their courtships and seeing them defending their territories at the top of the wall.

After a brief look around our new residence, we decided that it was time for a cup of tea, before we started to move some of our things into the wardrobe. It was not exactly a wardrobe, but definitely a sort of wardrobe. Everything seemed to be a sort of something, but not quite a finished anything. Still, they had had a devastating hurricane, so it was probably understandable. At least the bed looked reasonable. Maybe it *was* the finished article. We were just about to try it out, when the doorbell rang. We nearly jumped out of our socks. The last thing we had expected was a doorbell. It was Alua, looking pristine in her immaculate whites. "Tea is ready, if you are ready," she announced. We were ready. We had not eaten all day.

Inside the staff bungalow the whole of the hospital staff was drawn up in order of seniority, the staff on duty being dressed in white, the rest obviously dressed in their Sunday best. It was as warm and as cheerful a sight as one could hope to see. As soon as the introductions were over, it was as though a dam had burst. They were so warm and affectionate. Sue was the real centre of interest. How many children had we? "Come sit; we eat now." And with that, food was produced.

Have you ever tried eating spaghetti sandwiches? Until that moment, neither had we. It takes a lot of concentration. Despite my hunger, I eventually decided that one had to be born a Polynesian to acquire a taste for cold tinned spaghetti between two doorstep-sized slices of bread. The rest of the festive table consisted of corned beef and tinned pilchards. We had good appetites and did justice to their efforts, but we also bore in mind that we should leave enough for the nurses to take home to their families. Tinned food was not only expensive, but was also difficult to obtain. It was a treat for them, as well as being a first for us.

The morning dawned to the sound of many voices chirruping away outside our windows, like so many crickets. We later discovered that it was the duty of each small community to help keep the hospital grounds clean, tidy and free of weeds. This duty was, of course, delegated to the womenfolk.

We looked out of our window. It was a dream view, early in the morning. It was such a view as one sees in a Hollywood movie and which one knows is only achieved with fakery. The only view which could beat this picture of the Samoan sunrise was that from the same window at sunset. The hospital was truly built in a beautiful position. As we watched we saw a tall figure, dressed in a lava-lava and carrying a trident as he climbed carefully down the cliff to the sea. It could well have been Neptune, but it was just a local fisherman going off to catch his evening meal. Nothing could have been more perfect for the start of our new life, for our first morning on Savaii.

Behind us the ground rose steeply to the rim of the volcano, the source, as I had been told, of our water supply. The thought brought me down to earth. It was time for a cup of tea, and then – off to see what the Wizard of Oz had in store for me this time around.

Doctor in Residence (Samoan style)

The walk from our new quarters to the hospital produced cheery waves from our driver who was busy doing nothing, and many smiles from the crowded entrance hall. The matron, Alua, was there to greet me, a beam on her face and a fresh white uniform gracing her junoesque figure. Whilst showing me to what was to be my consulting room, she briefly explained the way that they, the nursing staff, had been used to dealing with the patients. It was little different to most practices back home in England. The patients would be sent in to me one at a time, usually with their records, if the nurse on reception had been able to find them. In a society in which people would regularly change their names, keeping track of their records was not always easy. Otherwise, the routine was very familiar to me. If the patient required a prescription, I would write it out and give it to the patient, who would go back to the window where he had picked up his records. He would hand it to the nurse together with a sum of money, which entitled him to his medication. There were few exemptions. If there was the need for minor surgery of any sort, then I would arrange it for when we had time and staff. I soon learned that there was not a great deal of difference between the medical complaints here and those I would see back in the U.K., even down to the excuses presented for being unable to work – a very interesting field of study and worthy of a thesis in its own right.

On this first morning in the hospital, I worked through the list until Alua came in with a welcome cup of tea. She informed me that the waiting room was now empty, so would I like to go round the wards to visit the in-patients. She had a bundle of records under her arm and it was obvious that she was ready. I soon learned that, although Alua was rather weak on medical knowledge, she was administratively very sound; she was a veritable mine of information. She knew every family, with intimate knowledge of the relations and the relationships. This knowledge she put to good use in deciding on admissions to the hospital. I soon learned that it was as well to ask her advice on all but medical matters.

As we went round the hospital, Alua gently eased me into the job and let me know what was expected of me. It seemed that one of my duties would be to make twice-weekly visits to two other clinics on the island. These were each about five miles from the hospital and were staffed by a nursing sister assisted by auxiliaries. If any operations were needed, the patients would be brought back to our hospital, where we had a delivery room and a minor operating theatre. The procedure at the clinics was similar to that at the main hospital, but with two differences. At least in the hospital at Sataua it was accepted that I was the boss. The nurses at the two clinics appeared to be a law unto themselves. That was bad enough, but what annoyed me even more was the state of clinics; they were filthy. Alua had no jurisdiction over them and simple nursing disciplines appeared to have been abandoned.

There was a second hospital on Savaii, at Palauli near the other end of the island, close to the ferry terminal. In fact it was that hospital, which we had visited on our first visit to Samoa five years earlier. It was well equipped, with a clean operating theatre. I was told that it was normally staffed by an elderly doctor, who was a trained obstetrician, together with a junior doctor as an assistant. Between them they managed to attend their hospital on two days out of seven. The rest of the time, they could be found – or more often not found – somewhere on the mainland. In fact, in all the time that we were on Savaii, I never set eyes on either one of them. It looked as if any doctoring to be done, would have to be done by me.

Every cloud has a silver lining – and there was one on Savaii. Terry Svensen's wife, Luanna, the former Miss World, came from a family which owned a large plot of land, with beach frontage, at Manase on the northern tip of Savaii. Through Terry's contacts, for he had done a lot of work for a firm which had built a hydro-electric dam on Upolu, he had acquired a large number of steel containers, which were no longer required after the completion of the contract. With a little cutting and welding, the containers were soon turned into very presentable little chalets. These were shipped over and installed on his wife's family land. Terry quickly had a small waterfront resort up and running. He hired the best cook on Samoa and 'bang', he was away. Everyone wanted to go there for the weekend; it was the most fashionable place in the South Pacific.

At our first meeting, Terry had asked me to sort out the rather dirty abscess on his leg. It had been troubling him for over three months and had become resistant to all the antibiotics available locally. I had managed to settle it down using medication from my own stock and, after that, Sue and I had been virtually welcomed into his family.

Upon learning of our posting to Savaii, he had instructed his staff to keep one of the chalets at Manase available for our use. It was his gift. If they were to need a doctor, would I be able to help them out, please? I suppose it was *quid pro quo* all round. We did not know when we would be able to take advantage of his offer, but we looked forward to a weekend of leisure, and we would only have to find the money for our food and drink.

The hospital water supply came from the mountains and fed into two very large concrete tanks. We were therefore very surprised to learn that water was only available between eight o'clock in the morning and four o'clock in the afternoon. The reason for the restriction was simple, and we should have realised it from our experience on Tokelau. The hospital buildings included a wash house block. No patient could miss the opportunity. It was not a case of bringing a toothbrush and an overnight bag, but rather the entire family's weekly wash! But 'Cleanliness is next to Godliness', so what could we say?

At this spot in the world, about as far away from anywhere as it was possible to get, it was rather a surprise to be awoken at 3 o'clock in the morning by the sound of a bus, with its venerable diesel engine. Not that I could hear the engine, for it was drowned out by the blaring of the radio and the driver singing at the top of his not inconsiderable voice. From Sataua it was a two hour drive to the wharf at Salelologa to meet the first boat from the mainland. I imagined the driver was lonely at that time of the night. There was no point in me getting up so early. There was no water and no 'telly'. Sue was snoring peacefully, completely oblivious of the arrival of the first bus, so I closed my eyes. I must have dozed off, for suddenly it was eight o'clock. Out of bed; a slice of toast; and then off to work.

On that second morning there were about 12 people waiting to see me. Instant diagnosis, instant treatment; and then across to the ward. I was very pleased that I was able to discharge most of the patients. It was amazing how many asthmatics were among them.

In the afternoon an elderly woman brought in a child of about two years old. Following behind was a girl of about sixteen. I quickly realised that these were grandmother, mother and child. They were not well. The mother was wheezing badly and the child, instead of looking a nice shade of brown, was a blue brown colour. Its eyes were bulging and its chest was hardly moving. It was another family of asthmatics. What in God's name was happening out here in the South Pacific? However, in one respect we *were* better off than on Tokelau. At least we had oxygen and we had a radio-telephone which was always available. We had something to offer to our patients.

On Fakaofo we had relied upon John and Neta as the source of all the latest news. The equivalent on Savaii was one of our nurses, Toy Eva, and her boyfriend, who was the captain of one of the ferries. Incidentally, I loved the name Toy Eva, it sounded so liquid and soft. What a pity then to learn that, translated into English, it meant 'Number Nine'! I imagine that, after the first eight, her parents had run out of names. But back to the news. What we were told was that all those administrators sent from New Zealand to Tokelau were to remain there and were to form the nucleus of a new government for the islanders. It seemed that the paymasters in N.Z. had at last figured out what had been going on, and where all the money had been going. I wondered if this might have had anything to do with us.

Some days later, I was surprised to see a familiar face approaching the hospital.

We had met Warren Joplin when we first visited Samoa in 1991. Now he was calling in at the hospital with a tour group, which he asked me to take round the hospital. Both Sue and I were delighted to see him and only too pleased to oblige. After the tour, Sue offered the group cups of tea and a chat about life on Savaii. This became a regular occurrence, with Warren making the hospital a routine stop on his tours. On occasions the tour members would reciprocate our hospitality by offering us sweets or chocolates. These were like birthday treats for Sue. As a chocoholic, she felt very sadly deprived of such luxuries. For the tour groups, it was an additional item of interest for them to discuss when they arrived back at their hotel.

Much as Sue enjoyed the chocolates, I think that she looked forward to these visits even more because they offered the opportunity of someone else to talk to. Also Warren had a very good library back at the hotel and he would bring us books.

He stayed at the Safua Hotel. It was not a modern building, but was made up of separate *fales*, constructed in the native style, with thatched straw roofs. During the night, one could listen as the termites munched their way through the roof, and in the morning one would be covered in their excreta. Primitive as were the facilities, there was at least running water, albeit intermittent, and each *fale* was fitted with a toilet.

As I became more familiar with the routine of the hospital, I found that I had cause to telephone Apia. There was a phone in the consulting room, but I was unable to get a dial tone. Strangely there seemed no problem in receiving incoming calls, so I enquired what was going on. I was informed that the previous Doctor had run up such a large bill in making private calls that the hospital authorities had refused to pay. As a result the telephone company had barred the telephone to outgoing calls. It was a major inconvenience as, in order to make a call, I had to send a radio-telephone message to the office in Apia. They, in turn would phone the person to whom I wished to speak, asking him to ring me at the hospital.

When we needed supplies, Sue and I would pay a visit to the Big Store (our co-operative), which was situated in the nearby village. There we could stock up with beers, Cokes and fruit juice. To get home we hitched a ride on the 'works bus', as I christened the local transport service. The bus went right around the island and we came to rely on it to get to the village and the stores. On that first occasion, we were not familiar with the routine, and just said, "Hospital, please." The driver not only let us on, but drove us right up to the hospital entrance before letting us off. He had a beaming smile on his face and wouldn't take any money. It seemed that news of our arrival had already spread.

Upon our departure from Tokelau, I had sworn never to eat another fish, but, like most resolutions, this one had little chance of success. Although there was a slightly greater variety of food available on Samoa, fish was still the staple diet. Anyway, we really enjoyed fish and when it was well prepared, with onion and some green beans, such as we had that evening, then it was delicious, especially when followed by some *esi* (pawpaw) as afters.

After the meal, Sue set about her evening exercise, big game hunting. She went round our quarters, spraying everything in sight. According to her, the idea was to frighten the cockroaches out into the open, when I should give chase and finish them off. That was not so easy; they were armour-plated. Sue had one big one in her sights and was spraying it like mad, until I pointed out that it was one that I had killed earlier and had just kicked out of the way. (No proper funeral. You got callous after a while!) Usually the ants would soon polish off any corpses, but they had obviously not yet found this one.

Before bed, I popped back across to the hospital, where one of the patients had bronchial trouble. She was rather a large lady and it was no time for delicacy. Everyone else in the ward thought it hilarious, as I beat the hell out of her chest. She seemed to enjoy it and so did I. It was not long before she was coughing up buckets of sputum. Now we could both get a good night's sleep.

The next morning, we were again awakened by the crickets, or rather by the early morning clean-up brigade. The women took it in turn to tidy up the hospital grounds, and they invariably started as soon as it was light. They sat on the volcanic cinders, which made up most of the ground, each cleaning and weeding her own little patch and chattering away as they worked. I suspected that it was more of a social get-together than a real working party. Anyway, we took the hint and also decided to make an early start. We had at least had the foresight to fill the kettle before we went to bed. We had already learned that if we got up too early, the night nurse may not have switched on the water pump, and I had not yet found out where the switch was hidden. I really regretted that I could not understand the Samoan language. I knew that the Samoans often understood us much better than they would admit, but if there was something they did not wish to divulge, then they hid the fact that they could understand, just as they had with Margaret Mead in the 1920s. My vocabulary was limited to a few odd words and the ability to mime, or, when necessary, a loud voice, with which to shout "Help!" that usually bought one or other of the staff running to my aid.

As we drank our cup of early morning tea, we watched as the children of the village came down to the beach and began filling bags with volcanic ash. We learned that most of the floors of the *fales* consisted simply of this powdered lava. There was no need to wash floors. It was easier simply to scatter a fresh layer of nice clean ash on top of the old layer!

Just as on Tokelau, we soon learned how thoughtful and generous the local people were. If someone had cooked a particular dish, which they thought that Sue and I might like, then they always brought us a bowl full. They tried to demonstrate their gratitude to us in many small ways.

In particular, there was one very short, very dumpy elderly lady. She was a sort of orderly, who helped out in the hospital. She was a general dog's-body, helping everyone and being everyone's grandma. She took a particular liking to Sue, partly, I think, because she had the same name, although she spelt it Soo. She immediately 'adopted' Sue and was forever bringing across special little titbits or local delicacies for her. She would then sit around as Sue told her about our children and showed her photographs of everyone. As for the treats she brought for us, we did once enquire as to what was in them, but found that the explanations were too much for our cultivated stomachs, so we soon stopped it. Once or twice we recognised that what she had brought us was chicken, but it was like no chicken we had ever eaten. We wondered about its diet, as we found its flesh so tough as to be almost impossible to eat. We supposed that, if they had to scratch among the lava flow for their food, then it was not surprising that the local chickens were decidedly stringy. When all else failed, we would slip the meat to the dog which had adopted us. He found it equally tough.

Time for a Break

We had finally reached the stage where we could allow ourselves a short break away from the hospital and, having been invited to Terry Svensen's beach resort, we had arranged that our driver would take us around the north of the island to Manase. We were going to have a rest.

Or so I thought, until we got underway. There was effectively only one road on Savaii and that went all around the island. At least the map showed it as going right around. However, the reality was that there was a stretch along the north coast which might generously be described as minor road. Unfortunately this stretch lay between Sataua and Manase. The drive was one of the most painful experiences which my backside had faced since I had had my haemorrhoids treated. The first twenty minutes of the drive were reasonable. The road was more or less covered in tarmac, with just a reasonable number of potholes to the square yard; but then we entered what seemed to be an earthquake disaster zone. If there was a road, then it was very well concealed and, to my untutored eye, invisible. It took us two hours of absolute hell to drive this short distance around the island. By the time we reached our destination, I had serious misgivings about the enterprise, but it turned out to be well worth the temporary discomfort.

The staff at Manase were very kind. The metal cabins were comfortably furnished and the food was good. To our great surprise, we discovered that the head chef was Adrianne, the lady whose restaurant had been burned down in Apia. We had heard that Terry Svensen had hired the best cook on Samoa and now we knew who it was.

The water in the lagoon was warm; Sue even got me out to the coral reef. This was really smart of her. She swims like a fish, and with the stamina of a fish, whereas I flounder like a flounder. Anyway, with me holding on to her waist and her doing all the work, we were able to make it to the reef. There we could view the coral and its inhabitants. It was spectacular, with the fishes varied and colourful in their beautiful setting. We were surprised how 'tame' the fish were, not at all upset by our presence. We later learned that Terry would swim out to the reef and hand feed them, which probably explained why they swarmed around us in such brilliant profusion.

Although we had not got a great deal of money to spend on food or drink, it was lovely to be looked after for a while.

On the Sunday morning Terry's wife, Luanna, took us to meet her family and also took the opportunity to ask me to diagnose an ailment affecting one member of the family. Then we all went off together to look at the little hospital-cum-dressing-station that had been built in the village. They had a part-time nursing aid looking after it, mainly, we gathered, to ensure that not too much of the equipment was stolen. An interesting discussion ensued between Terry and Luanna and her family. Terry had it in mind to purchase the little clinic and to turn it into a private hospital. It was only at this point that I realised the underlying purpose of our visit. Terry turned to me and asked whether I would be interested in running the hospital. I would not need to worry about anything; he would square it with the Prime Minister.

It was an interesting proposition. Certainly life would have been much more comfortable for us. We would have been able to live in Manase and have our meals either there or with Luanna's family, all very cosy. I had no doubt that Terry would grasp the chance to advertise his Manase as having its own qualified medical officer. He was a great guy was Terry, but he never missed a trick. For my part, I had to consider the other islanders. They would not have benefited from such a move and, with some reluctance, I had to decline the offer.

We called in to look at a patient of the local nurse and then it was time for our drive back to Sataua. All good things had to come to an end. The weekend had been so pleasant and relaxing that I did not even notice the discomfort of the return journey.

Life went on and, before we knew it, it was the end of May. At 6.30 in the evening we had just arrived back from visiting the outlying clinics. We had left at 8.30 in the morning and, after seeing about 20 patients at Foailalo, we had set off on a further two hour drive to the hospital at Palauli. We were told that the other two Doctors had left as soon as they learned that I had arrived at Sataua, leaving me as the only Doctor on Savaii. Therefore the nurse had called me to look at a patient whose condition was causing her concern. While I was there I was asked to see more outpatients and a ward full of in-patients. Then it was off to the police station. A little girl had been killed in a road accident on the previous Friday. I was told that the body had been accidentally (?) released and buried on the Saturday and now the police wanted to prosecute the driver. My job would be to read the hospital notes and decide how and why the child had died. A post-mortem without a body; it was a first for me. But then, this was the South Pacific.

Back at the fort, or more precisely the hospital at Sataua, the atmosphere was alive with rumours. Alua had been away attending an administrative course on the main island and had discovered that the other parts of Savaii were in rebellious mood. They were not happy that the *papalagi* doctor was spending so much time at Sataua and so little at the other medical centres. It seemed that, more often than not, I was the only doctor on the island, ministering to a population of 45,000 people. I did not know whether to be flattered or annoyed. It was good to be appreciated, but I felt that there was a limit to the amount of territory I could cover.

Sometimes we had to smile. There were we, trying to survive on Sue's budget, based on the principle of 'South Pacific on $5 a day', with me a pensioner and Sue an unemployed administrator, and yet we were perceived as these affluent *papalagi*. One of the assistant nurses tried to tap me for a loan, but I had to tell her that I had lent the last of my money to our driver. If she were able to get the ten dollars back from him, then she could borrow it! I don't know if she was successful, but, if so, she would almost certainly have lent the money to someone else. I didn't know if anyone had any real money. The government was notoriously slow at paying bills or salaries. It didn't seem to matter anyway; the Samoan motto was 'what's yours is mine' – and sometimes vice versa.

The trip to Palauli hospital was becoming a regular part of my routine, but on one occasion our transport finally died; not of shame, but simply of old age and exhaustion. It had undergone just too many makeshift repairs, using parts from even older irreparable vehicles. The Pacific islands were full of such vehicles. They were already junk when they were imported from unscrupulous dealers in America or Japan. Our rust bucket had been dying for a long time. Even the tyres were historical relics, consisting mainly of the canvas linings with hardly any evidence of them ever having been coated in rubber. It was only the indomitable will of our driver that had kept it on the road for so long – plus the fact that he did not get paid unless the vehicle was mobile. Anyway, on this occasion, the universal joint, whatever that might be, had given up the ghost. Another passing mobile wreck towed us to Foailalo hospital, where the real fun began. Foailalo hospital had the luxury of a Transport Manager. Surely he could manage to find us a vehicle to take us back to Sataua? Oh, no; nothing as simple as that. Instead he sent a car to Salelologa to find the minister responsible for transport on the entire island and to enquire whether he might provide us with a vehicle. Then having received the go-ahead, he sent the car 120 kilometres anti-clockwise around the north coast of the island, to pick us up and then to continue all the way back home over the same extended route in the same anti-clockwise direction. I never figured it out, unless the driver was paid by the mile, or maybe he just enjoyed the sensation of the ruts and potholes between Manase and Sataua. He had effectively driven twice around the island to get us from Foailalo to Sataua, which were approximately 30 kilometres apart.

When we finally got back to base, we found an invitation awaiting us. Sue and I were invited to lunch with the Minister of Health, the Hon. Sala Vaimili II and Mrs. Vaimili II the following day. When we arrived we found that the reception was to welcome a certain Dr. and Mrs. White. We eventually discovered that he was a cardiologist from New Zealand, but we never found out why he was being honoured in this way. In a long-winded speech, during which, in accordance with Samoan tradition, every point was repeated in a number of different ways, the minister expressed his gratitude on behalf of the people of Samoa. Eventually we sat down to eat and I must admit it was a good meal. Then there was a further presentation ceremony during which a title was conferred upon Dr. White. I decided that he must have done something very significant for Samoa in the past.

From what we had heard of the state's economy, we were not sure how the government would manage to pay for this celebratory meal, but, as one of the government ministers owned the hotel, we assumed that somehow it would be settled. In fact, while speaking to the minister after the meal, he admitted to me that, on the previous Tuesday, the government had had just 53 tala (Samoan dollars) in the kitty. Fortunately he did not try to tap me for a loan, or I would have had to refer him to the assistant nurse at the hospital! The Samoan rate of exchange was completely artificial. Officially the rate stood at three tala to the pound, but outside Samoa the currency was worth virtually nothing.

The minister expressed his gratitude for the work we were doing and passed on the personal appreciation of the Prime Minister. Furthermore, he intimated that they might be able to offer me a fresh contract to enable me to stay for a further year. I managed to keep a straight face and to thank him in an appropriate fashion.

As to our replacement transport, no commitment was forthcoming. I had my doubts.

Crises in Casualty

By 5 o'clock we were back at the hospital, but had not even had time for a cup of tea when Alua sent over to ask if I could come across to the hospital. She said that they had admitted a patient who had dislocated his shoulder playing rugby. I strolled over to the casualty area, where quite a crowd had gathered. Alua had already assured them that the clever doctor would quickly reset his shoulder. God forgive her! It was obvious that the poor fellow's neck was fractured. I sent everyone off with whatever bags and pillowcases I could find, telling them to fill them with sand. By now the patient had realised the gravity of his situation. The last player who had suffered a similar injury had not survived for long. He cried out for a priest. When the priest turned up, he took one look at the patient, turned on his heel, said, "He's not one of mine," and walked off.

I eventually managed to push through the throng to insert an intravenous drip into the patient and to support his head and neck with sandbags. It was a Saturday and there would be no ferry until Monday, but it was crucial to get him to Apia. We would have to move him from our hospital down to the wharf, which was a two-hour-drive away at the other end of the island and then somehow get him on to a boat to take him to the main hospital in Apia. Our own vehicle was 'dead' – and it was obvious that everyone expected our patient to be in a similar condition in the very near future. I was not so certain. Although he was paralysed from the neck down, he was breathing well and his heart rate was stable, as, even more surprisingly, was his blood pressure.

Our casualty room was getting fuller. Everyone from the village wanted a piece of the action. I supposed that, with no TV or radio, this was their nearest equivalent to Emergency Ward 10, or Dr. Finlay's Casebook. However, the mass of bodies did not make my job any easier. The trickiest bit would be to get the patient off the table and on to a solid stretcher. We then had to get him into, or onto, a vehicle (as yet unidentified) and then to the hospital at Palauli. There he would rest until Monday, when he would be driven the last few miles to Salelologa and the ferry. Once on the main island of Upolu, there would be the further drive to the hospital in Apia. The logistics were daunting – and yet somehow we had to do it, and do it without killing the patient.

Eventually we found someone with a flat truck and slowly we lifted the patient on to it. I couldn't imagine how he was going to cope with the ride along the south of the island, let alone the boat ride across the strait to Faleolo, which would take a good hour, with a further hour's drive to the hospital.

By the Monday evening we knew that we had succeeded. The man was now in the main hospital and his condition was still stable. We had done our best. Whether we had really done him any favours was a more difficult question, but he was still alive when we finally left Samoa some months later.

I have mentioned the problems caused by the number of 'spectators' jamming the ward while we were treating the patient. This situation was exacerbated, when, while all this was taking place, an old man in the next ward decided to have a heart attack. We only had one bottle of oxygen in the hospital and that was being used to treat the patient with the broken neck. Somehow we had to get the old man through the throng and into the casualty ward. With so many people in the way and the two sets of relatives each crying for priority, it was like a French farce. Eventually we got the old man on to a makeshift bed in the treatment room, but with all the relatives crowding around, I found it impossible to get near him. It was only when his condition was clearly deteriorating and he was having difficulty in breathing, that they moved out of the way, saying "Come on. Get on and make him better." I just hoped that our oxygen supply was going to last out, as both patients were going to need it. The heat, the noise and the congestion were indescribable. It was worse than Piccadilly Station. It was absolutely essential to get the villagers out of the room, so that we had room to work. Even then, they would not disperse and every window had a crowd of faces peering in. At last everything settled down; the one patient was sent off to Palauli and the old man's condition stabilised. After a week of careful nursing, he was able to go home to his family.

We were just beginning to think that we had settled down to a comfortable routine, when things began to go wrong. We had learnt to live without a telephone and we were getting used to being stranded at Sataua, due to the lack of transport. However, now we had no running water and the power had failed. I thought that maybe we should devote the day to prayer. Our fridge/freezer was beginning to warm up, so everything we had kept so carefully was going to be ruined. To make things even worse, we could get no answer on the radio link. Yes, prayer would be the best thing.

That evening we sat down to relax, in the certain knowledge that nothing else could go wrong. Everything electrical, mechanical or hydraulic had already ceased to function, or so we thought. We were sitting listening to our little tape player when it developed a fault. It must have been the loudspeaker, as it still worked on the earpiece. It was only a little thing, but for us it was a major disappointment; quite apart from the fact that, by the time we got home, the guarantee would have run out.

The one bright spot was an invitation to lunch with the local M.P., who had introduced himself to us simply as Fritz. We found ourselves seated next to him at the top table. He voiced his pleasure at our work and said that he thought I would be offered a fresh year's contract in September. I smiled and expressed my gratitude and tried to be pleasant to everyone. The M.P. asked if I would write him a paper on what was needed to make the hospitals fit the aspirations of the people. He really meant the dressing stations, but he was not alone in insisting on calling them hospitals. Even in the coloured brochures advertising Samoa, they boasted about the number of hospitals they had. Anyway, I promised him that I would write him a paper as he had asked. He then kindly offered us free accommodation in his hotel. It turned out that he owned one of the large hotels in Apia. I just hoped that we could take advantage of his offer before it was time for us to leave. The first beer would be free; after that we would have to pay. While I had been talking to the M.P., Sue had struck up conversation with another *papalagi*, who came from Guisley near Leeds, not more than 20 miles from our home in England – almost a blood relation, one might say. At the end of the reception, the M.P. arranged an ambulance to take us back to Sataua. It had been an interesting day. I was beginning to look forward to Saturdays; there was always something interesting happening on Saturday.

This thought had only just crossed my mind, when something happened to make me reconsider. Rather than just an 'interesting Saturday', the day became known as the 'Day of the Big Accident'.

It all began when the headmaster of our big school took his wife and pregnant daughter-in-law out shopping for the week's groceries. There were two general stores, one of them belonging to a relative of the headmaster's wife, and the other belonging to a Chinese merchant. The Chinese store was considerably cheaper than that of the relative, which resulted in an argument each week as to which store they should patronise. On that particular afternoon, the headmaster had picked up a bottle of spirits from the store and had gone back to his car, where he had sat drinking. Shopping offered the major opportunity to meet old friends and to exchange news and gossip. This all took considerable time and, in that time, one could make a considerable impression on a bottle of spirits, at the same time working up a fair head of steam. By the time the two women returned to the car, with the son carrying the shopping, the headmaster was just about ready to explode, so a first class argument ensued. He just had time to finish off the last of the spirits, before driving off with the family. The road was twisty and, going downhill, he had run out of road and rolled the car.

When they arrived at the hospital, I could see that the headmaster had more or less scalped himself, and he had neatly severed the muscles at the back of his lower left leg, literally down to the bone. His wife had a fracture of the right forearm and her shoulder was dislocated, but otherwise, apart from being shocked, she seemed satisfactory. I could not find anything wrong with the pregnant woman, which was amazing, but wonderful. I was not sure what we could have done for her, as equipment in the hospital was virtually nil. It was hardly better than on Tokelau.

I pulled the fractured forearm straight, and left Sue with the other nurse to deal with the plastering, while I started stitching up the headmaster. We had no anaesthetics to give him, as, once again, we had a hospital with no supplies. Nothing had been replaced since the cyclone. Fortunately he was so drunk that he didn't need our help.

Sue was having problems with the plaster of Paris. It was so old that it would not set. Meanwhile I had started on the headmaster's head. It truly looked as if he had been scalped by Red Indians. Our examination couch was small and this man was a typical Samoan, so he hung over the sides. I was just a little concerned that he would start to move and fall off. Fortunately the drink had kicked in and he lay as in a coma.

By this time, word had started to spread around the village. The people on our side of the island had no access to radio or television. Apart from occasional facilities provided by some of the 15 religions on the island, all entertainment had to be home-made. Any unusual activity at the hospital became an instant attraction. Also, as everyone claimed to be related to everyone else, they all claimed the right to be there. Those who managed to squeeze into our small examination room strained for a good view and then fed back a running commentary to those behind them. The window seats were the most favoured locations, as these provided a good view from outside. Where treatment was extended, such as on this occasion, the locals would even bring along their coconut and cooked fish and have an impromptu picnic. Our staff, however hard they tried, could not get them away. It was like a wave, with pressure from the back pushing in, and our staff valiantly pushing them back. It was difficult for us to treat the patients properly, with people crushing in on us so closely. Sometimes, if we were lucky and the patient looked sufficiently moribund, they would back off and leave a little working space. It was as if they thought that it was only when the patient was close to death that he offered enough of a challenge. (In fact, they would even bring in patients who had obviously given up the struggle to live some considerable time before, and would demand that we perform medicine magic to restore them.)

I had soon run out of catgut for stitching the muscles, so I had to cobbled them together as best I could. Then, with Sue holding the leg together, I started on the skin. Alua said, "We have no more stuff for the leg. You used all of it on his head," as though I had done it deliberately. I sent Sue off to get a bobbin of white sewing thread. It was fortunate that she had brought a sewing kit with her. We boiled it up with a little antiseptic, just to show that there was no ill-feeling.

In the meantime, Sue and the nurse, by a dint of trial and error, had managed to get a plaster on to the poor woman's arm and they were able to turn their attention to assist me with the headmaster. His blood pressure had started to fall. He had, after all, lost a lot of the red stuff. Poor Sue! She knew, of course, what was coming. As I have mentioned before, she was my walking blood bank. She is one of those wonderful people whose blood group is such that their blood is compatible with all other groups. She is a universal donor, whose blood can be given to anyone. The audience were really getting their money's worth at this show. A pint of Sue's white Anglo-Saxon female blood soon had the headmaster safe and sound, not that he showed any concern about it. He had snored his way through the entire procedure. We never found out what he had drunk, or how much, but, as an anaesthetic, it had been very effective.

The headmaster recovered from his injuries, but I doubt whether he ever got over the story of the accident or the treatment received at the hospital. The story had reached Apia long before he did, forever after, he was the man who was saved by the blood of that little *papalagi* woman. His leg was pulled unmercifully. It seems that, had he been conscious, he would have refused to accept the blood of a woman, particularly that of a white woman. It flew in the face of their custom and tradition. However, I'm sure he would not have survived without it. As it was, it all turned out well. He made a full recovery. His wife's fractured arm healed with the bone more or less in line. The son was fine and the pregnant daughter had no lasting ill effects. However, after we had carried out emergency treatment, they were all taken to Apia hospital for monitoring until their injuries healed.

A Foreign Invasion

We were still chuckling about the incident with the headmaster, when another opportunity arose, not for me this time, but for Sue. She was asked by the nurses if she would like to go with them out on district.

It had been arranged that a vehicle would come over from the main island, with a driver, and they would tour the island, checking every hill and dale, looking for even the smallest community in order to follow up a child welfare and vaccination programme funded by the World Health Organisation. It was hard work, but it was right up Sue's street!

The team would leave at six in the morning and would often be away for 12 or 13 hours. Once or twice Sue took the camcorder and took some wonderful film. They would travel out into the hills, sometimes leaving the van and hiking up the track to find a family, taking with them a small box of equipment. If the family were not at home, they may have to follow them for miles; maybe they had gone to visit a friend, or just gone walk-about. It was no wonder that the nurses were exhausted when they eventually arrived back at the hospital. Sue was certainly very weary. In contrast, my life was relatively relaxed, as we still had no transport, so were unable to visit any of the other 'hospitals'.

Eventually this situation came to an end and, at 6 o'clock one morning, an ambulance arrived to take Sue and me off to visit every hospital and dressing station on Savaii. Apparently the authorities had finally reacted to popular demand. We were impressed – and at least the ambulance had comfortable seats. As the day progressed, we visited the various dressing stations and at each one we were offered food. It seemed that the doctor responsible for looking after the eastern end of the island had not been seen for days; maybe he was on holiday. No one was sure; there was no telephone.

It was about midnight when we were awoken again. "Hospital, transport; you come. Other hospital; you go!" That was all the information we could get out of the driver. Perhaps it was just as well. There was no lighting on the road, but that was normal. However, as we approached the hospital at Palauli we realised that that too was in total darkness. That was not so normal.

A torchbearer led us into the ward and a nurse just said, "She dying." Sometimes one was assumed to be a mind-reader. After explaining to us that there were no lights, which was pretty obvious, the nurse eventually agreed to let us see the patient, so as to make our own diagnosis. Some details of the patient would be more useful than a whole lot of uninformed opinion. At last we got the story. The woman had been delivered of a full-term baby earlier in the day, but had continued bleeding long after the birth. "Not so much now," added the nurse helpfully. Not only was this self evident, but was to be expected. She had clearly lost a lot of blood. The first thing was to set up an intravenous drip. However, I could see no blood vessel in which to insert the transfusion needle, so I would have to cut into her ankle to find one. This is a relatively simple procedure, except in virtual darkness. With Sue holding the torch and me juggling my spectacles and the instruments, we eventually got a drip going. At last I was able to examine the poor patient. She had been torn during her delivery and, as soon as I was able to transfer my attention to this and put in some stitches, then all was well. She would make a good recovery.

It did not seem quite so dark on the drive back home. We were too tired to make ourselves even a cup of tea, so we fell straight into bed. It would soon be morning and time to start another day's work.

While Sue was off with the nurses, spending another day visiting what I referred to as 'the Plantations', Alua came in to tell me of the imminent arrival of a boatload of Americans. "What is it, tourists?" I asked. "No, Christian Aid workers." "What in heaven's name can they do for us?" Alua didn't know, but, "The last time they came, the villagers all got spectacles." I just could not believe it. Then I was informed that they were to have the run of the hospital. My spirits bucked up. Perhaps they *would* be able to help. We urgently needed a building team. The entire hospital was just as the hurricane had left it.

Therefore with some expectation I waited to meet them the following morning. I was totally ignored. By 10 o'clock the hospital was full of earnest young men and women, setting up clinics in every spare corner. Prayer meetings and counselling sessions were in full swing, and sackloads of spectacles were being emptied on to tables. The rest of the hospital was filling with people clamouring with their own particular demands. There was even a man with a wooden leg, who had heard that the Americans had brought some of the smart new lightweight artificial legs.

There was no room for me in this massive Church revival. They may have heard that I was not a Christian.

During the whole period of their stay, neither Sue nor I were ever invited on board their boat for a meal, although they were so gracious as to leave a few of their sandwiches for us at the hospital.

There was a more positive aspect to this American influx and this arrived in the shape of their Chief Engineer. His name, or rather his initials, were J.C., and a J.C. he turned out to be. We had a water steriliser, but it had never worked. J.C. got it going. Better still, he was able to show me how the whole contraption worked. He also offered to look at our cassette recorder and, after a bit of fiddling about with its internals, got the loudspeaker working again. For these, and many other small deeds, I forgave the other idiots and praised his name, or rather his initials.

By 7 o'clock the next morning, the villagers were queuing outside the hospital, waiting for whatever they could get for nothing. The aid team from the boat eventually turned up at 10 o'clock. I was so fed up, that I asked them to start the clinics on time. After all, the people had been told to get there by 8.30 a.m. All I received in response was, "We have to get our breakfast first." They spent the first part of the morning looking into people's eyes and then giving out glasses. Anyone who was fast enough could get two pairs, by joining the queue again.

I bumped into Soo, our nurse aid, or more precisely she bumped into me. She was wearing her new glasses. I asked her if she needed them. "No," she said, "but they were free. I get a pair each time they come. Eventually they start to hurt my eyes, so I put them with all the other pairs I have."

At lunchtime, the ophthalmic team managed to cause a mini riot. They decided to pack up while there were still about 20 people waiting to be given free spectacles, together with a few waiting to have them changed for a better class of headache! The team was obviously working on American time, rather than Samoan or Tokelauan time. After all, it was their lunchtime! Later they even offered me a couple of their left over sandwiches. I ran across to share them with Sue. They were chicken. We ate them slowly, savouring each and every mouthful. The chicken melted in our mouths like butter. That was the nearest we came to an invitation to their boat for a meal, although we did hear of others who had made it.

I received a visit from the ship's engineer, accompanied by one of our useless young men from the Samoan Public Health Department. They went up to take a look at the hospital water pump. Unfortunately even J.C was unable to do anything for it and pronounced it beyond repair. It was back to square one.

There was a doctor on board the ship, who addressed my staff the following day. He lectured them as though they were simple-minded five-year-olds. The young man from the Public Health Department translated for him, but didn't know any of the correct medical terms, so our staff spent most of the time giggling. I was so pleased when they left and I could get back to seeing to my patients. The only one of them worth his salt had been J.C. He could have been so useful to us. It was a pity he had to go off with the boat. Before they left, they off-loaded some medication for us. Most of it was not worth house room, just bottles and bottles of out-of-date cough mixture. (The one thing I had not required, during the six months we had been in the South Pacific, had been cough mixture.) Once the 'Mercy Ship' had gone, we began to get back to normal, or to what passed as normal on Savaii.

All Good, Clean, Healthy Fun

Sue had some exciting news. She had learned that there was a woman in the village who sold home-baked bread. We quickly decided to go for a walk, remembering to take some money with us. It was to no avail. She had sold out. However, she did promise to keep a loaf for us the following day. Anyway, it was a nice walk. All the locals thought that we were mad, going off for walks during the heat of the day, but that was when I felt at my best.

When we arrived back at the hospital, Alua struck up a conversation. She was in a chatty mood. She had been attending yet another meeting, at which she had heard that I was the only doctor for about 45,000 inhabitants. I thought that that was probably an exaggeration. She went on that the other hospitals were again demanding that I spend more time with them. She singled out Safotu hospital for special mention. Safotu was the hospital we had visited while on our trip to Svensen's resort at Manase, and was where Luanna's family lived. Oh yes, one could smell the intrigue! Either Terry or Luanna had been having words in high places.

Did we want the good news, or the bad news? Our driver was happy to give us both. A new vehicle had been allocated to us. It had been paid for by some or other international organisation. Unfortunately it had been commandeered by the main hospital in Apia, so we would not be getting it after all. Now the good news, they were sending us some tyres for our old wreck!

So we just waited, and carried on borrowing vehicles from wherever we could find them. Our best source was Iufi. She was our Staff Nurse, who was married to a young German lad. In fact, she had received her nursing training in Germany, so I had complete faith in her competence. What made her even more valuable was the fact that they owned a VW Combi, which was in excellent condition. For a consideration they would allow us to use it as an ambulance, provided that the patient was not too dirty! We would only use Iufi's vehicle if we had a really ill patient. Otherwise we would try to hire a pick up. We would put a couple of mattresses into the back and place the patient on top. The relatives and 'spectators' would then fill whatever space they could find. At least they were useful for holding up the drip sets on the journey back to the hospital.

During the short time we had been on Savaii, we had struck up an acquaintance with the lads working for the saw mill company. In particular, we had become friendly with Ian, a New Zealander, who was married to a Samoan girl. I had actually delivered their last child. The employees of the timber company lived in a special compound, which had its own beach frontage, just along the coast from the hospital. It was a lovely beach and very clean, so we jumped at an invitation to spend a day there. During the afternoon we had two power failures and in the evening we ended up reading by the light of paraffin lamps. At least it encouraged us to have an early night. This turned out to be fortuitous, as at least I was able to get a little sleep before I was roused at midnight to attend an emergency in the relocated labour ward. It was a delayed second stage delivery. I applied forceps and delivered the baby easily, but it was in white asphyxia and all attempts at resuscitation failed. It did not help that our oxygen cylinder was empty. The nurse was adamant that the patient had only arrived an hour previously. I was not so sure, but as she spoke no English, I could get no more information. I was devastated; it was the first baby that I had ever lost. To save trouble for everyone, and a mass of paperwork, I set it down as a still birth.

A couple of days later we had a visit from Warren. He brought us not only cooking utensils, but also some fresh vegetables as a gift from Moelagi Jackson. We explained our difficulties in contacting him and why we had not been in touch. The hospital authorities had still not paid the outstanding telephone bill, so our only means of communication was the radio transmitter. Even this was useless if there was no one at the other end to answer it. We thanked him for the vegetables, which were most welcome, and were sorry when he had to rush off. He had so much work that, in his words, the work was now running him.

Alua came in to inform us that there was an urgent radio message. Unfortunately the transmission had been badly broken up and all she had been able to understand was that there was a 4½-year-old child, with a temperature of 39°C and a rash. We had no transport, so I asked Alua to keep transmitting the message that the parents should bring the child to the hospital. They arrived about five hours later. It turned out to be a case of typhoid. The child came from the other end of the island, where the water supply was heavily polluted. I only realised this much later, when I observed that most typhoid cases seemed to come from that area.

I have previously mentioned the young man from the Public Health Department. He was one of a team who regularly visited the hospital. I had never seen any of them do a jot of work. When I mentioned the typhoid cases to them, they denied that there were any cases. I referred them to the case notes of the patients affected, but they simply said that these must have been incorrect diagnoses. "What?" I said, "all one hundred cases, seen and diagnosed by otherwise competent Samoan doctors?" The truth of the matter was that, if they acknowledge the presence of typhoid, they would have had to do something about it. The clinicians continued to diagnose the condition and the government laboratory, by using the wrong culture media, would continue to deny its existence. So the doctors kept on treating patients for an infection they did not have – and making them better, more or less. And the Public Health team just kept on drawing their salaries!

None of this should have surprised us. We had heard that the Minister of Health had no medical knowledge at all. In fact he had had very little education. He just happened to be a relative of a more powerful member of the government. Previously he had been running errands for one of the hotels. On the other hand, is that so different to what happens back in the U.K.? When I gave the matter a little more thought, I wondered whether, with his background, he might have been able to get us some carrier pigeons!

It is strange how you can see or hear something, sometimes quite regularly, and yet be completely unaware of it. Such a case was that of the Phantom Trumpet Blower. One evening I suddenly sat up and said to Sue, "Who's that blowing a horn?" She didn't know either, so next day we asked one of the nurses. She told us that it was a conch shell and it was blown every evening at sunset to warn people it was time to get off the roads and go home. Every Samoan knew that there were evil spirits just waiting for the darkness to waylay any unsuspecting villager. Better get home quickly! We must have heard it every evening since we arrived and yet we had never noticed it before. It was definitely not something we were used to in Pontefract.

A week later we were able to get off for another weekend at Manase. I informed Alua that we were going off for a dirty weekend, received with a knowing smile, and, after a quick round of the wards, we were on our way. Terry and Luanna were not there, but Luanna had left a package of fresh food for us. When it came time for us to leave, we found that their cash machine was not working, so, as we had no real money and I had picked up a bottle of Vodka at cost price from the bar, we got off very lightly.

When we arrived back home, Alua informed me that the following day she would be off to a committee meeting. That should be jolly.

Altogether it was a jolly day; I was beginning to feel like a vampire. Sue had to give blood again. The maternity cases only arrived at the hospital when they were in real trouble. I wondered what the true death rate in pregnancy and childbirth might be in Samoa. The published figures were purely fictitious. Dr. Bolinson of the World Health Organisation really hadn't got a clue.

Warren called in again, this time with an American tour group. He kindly brought us some beer, pineapple, tomatoes and books. What a good fellow he was. He told us of a plan for a BBC travel programme, in which he was to participate. What a pity that Steve and Ava could not get a similar boost for their new eco-tourism business.

It was Tuesday 14th June and we had had no running water since the Sunday. I tried to find out the reason, but it was as difficult as finding the lost chord. They were saying that it was due to a shortage of diesel fuel, but I knew that that was codswallop. There was plenty of fuel down at the ferry terminal at Salelologa. Not only had Iufi made some enquiries, but her husband had taken us down to see for ourselves. The visit was ostensibly to deliver our order for drugs, but we took the opportunity to make other enquiries. When we reached the office, we found that no staff were available. They were all at meetings. That seemed to be the way of things; never any work done, but plenty of time for meetings and for paperwork to be filled in. I said we would go off for a beer until the meeting was over, but then wanted action. When we returned a couple of hours later, I really tore into them. I told them that, if the diesel water pump was not working by the end of the day, then I was closing the hospital down. Furthermore, I would inform the Prime Minister, who had personally appointed me, and would advise Dr. Bolinson of the W.H.O., explaining why I was taking this action and who, in my opinion, was to blame for the situation.

After this little bit of fun, we drove round to Warren's place; I needed some replacement batteries for our Glucose meter. As usual, he organised it. It seemed that there were none of the correct batteries on Samoa, so he rang his brother in Australia; no trouble at all!

We arrived back home in time for supper – and to prepare another gourmet meal for the following day. We had been given a scrawny lump of chicken and a piece of pork. We mixed this up with a little of everything we had in the way of spices, onion, garlic, ginger, sugar and soya, and added some curry powder to finish it off. We left this little lot to marinade overnight in the refrigerator and cooked it the following morning with some taro.

I found it strange, how most births appeared to occur during the night. This night was no exception. Alua had delivered the baby, using her midwifery skills and a large pair of scissors. I thought that the local pork butcher had been at work. It took me nearly two hours to tidy the patient up, but not a moan from her. It was, after all, a male child.

By the following day, the water pump was back on line. Other than that it was a normal day, except of course, for the anticipation of our chicken and pork supper. It tasted ….. well, let me just say that the highlight of the meal was a small piece of Luanna's blue cheese. Now, that was real luxury!

The following morning, we missed the sound of the early bus. In fact there were no buses that day. Alua said it was due to the fact that there was no diesel or gasoline. The Transport Manager had forgotten to order any. Toy Eva chipped in that that was a normal state of affairs, and she should know, as her partner was skipper of one of the ferries. Toy Eva scared me, despite her liquid name! Her knowledge of nursing was minimal, but her confidence was tremendous, not only in her nursing skills, but also in her ability to attract men like moths around a flame. I was glad that Sue was usually close at hand.

We were in desperate need of milk donors, but there were no offers. Sue was close to losing her temper. She, an outsider, had given so freely of her blood and yet, when it came to a request for some breast milk, not one of the many mothers who had recently given birth was prepared to oblige. Eventually Sue struck lucky. She remembered the Samoan wife of the New Zealander, whom we had visited at the sawmill complex. At least there was one enlightened lady in the community.

There was one impoverished young family in the community that was causing me real concern, so much so that I admitted them into the hospital. They were undernourished and the baby would benefit from being cleaned and pampered. This decision did not find favour with the Women's Committee. They felt that the husband should pay for his stay in hospital. I hurriedly reassessed my diagnosis and admitted him as an emergency. His abdominal rumblings warranted further investigation… as soon as I could get around to it! The Committee were still not happy about it, but damn them, I was the boss and I was adamant; he was my emergency for the day.

We had begun to extend our walks in and around the village and, on one of our strolls we met up with the local head of the Catholic Church. We had quite a lengthy talk. He wanted to know why we did not attend church on Sundays – obviously our every move was being observed and reported. I explained that the hospital was my church and that the people in the hospital were my congregation and under my wing. He was getting a bit flustered, so I slipped in the bit about the source of the blood which had saved the headmaster, the food which was sustaining another of the villagers and the breast milk, without which one of his youngest parishioners may well have died. Gradually the light began dawning upon him. "These are very lazy and ignorant people," he said. We parted on the best of terms. I felt certain that he now had a new parable to relay to his flock, the best morality story in Samoa.

A couple of days later I caught Alua at it again. I would have to throw those infernal scissors away. She was a menace with them. She loved doing episiotomies (making an incision to assist childbirth.) This is a useful procedure when warranted, but the Samoan women rarely had complications sufficient to justify this intervention. They generally delivered their babies quite naturally and easily. Alua had obviously been shown how to perform this minor operation, but I felt that she must have had an ulterior motive for using it so often. Anyway the present patient was another example of her work, and now she was left with a cut – and what a savage cut. Thank goodness I was able to do a good repair job and stitch her up neatly.

I was chatting away to old Soo, when she came up with an interesting remark. "All *papalagis* smell," she said. I was intrigued. Most of the *papalagis* I knew washed and showered two or three times a day and used deodorants, whereas most of the Samoans did not bathe from one year's end to the next. And yet, according to Soo, it was we who smelled. I wondered whether it was the fact that we ate so much meat in our diet and thus smelled of beef and pork and mutton. The people of the Indian sub-continent love spices in their food. The South Pacific islanders on the other hand lived mainly on fish, and rarely added spices to their meals. The Tokelauans in the evening would sit in the sea and, while washing themselves and exchanging chit-chat, would grab a passing fish and just bite into it. That was their supper. I surmised that different places and different habits would result in different body odours.

Our cooking was certainly different to that of the locals. It was interesting to see Iufi's face when I gave her a taste of my fish patty. I showed her how I made it, with cooked tuna, spices and coconut milk. She had never thought of cooking fish like that. I also showed her how I cooked 'tuna sweet & sour'. Her husband thought that it was wonderful, just like his mother used to make back home in Germany. Iufi was back the next day to reciprocate. She brought us some of her tuna. She had pickled it in coconut milk and coconut cream. It was delicious, rather reminiscent of pickled herring. It went down very well with our home pickled onion and cucumber. Incidentally her husband had started a nice little business. He would collect local shells, clean and polish them, and then send them back to Germany, where there was a ready market. Between them, Iufi and her husband were doing sufficiently well to send the two children to school in New Zealand.

Saturday afternoon was the needlework class, particularly if there had been a rugby match. On this particular occasion, the local team had been beaten and the winners had to drive through our area on the way home. The losing team were waiting for them and, in a well-planned ambush, subjected them to a hail of stones, rocks and anything else which could be hurled in their direction. It was all good-natured, of course, as indicated by the verbal encouragement which accompanied the assault. We collected those who had been unsuccessful in evading this display of local patriotism and stitched them up. It was all good, clean, healthy fun!

We were still smiling about this, when one of our drivers was brought in, rather the worse for wear. His story was even better then that of the rugby players.

It appears that the driver was incensed that his neighbour's pigs had strayed onto his plantation and were destroying his crops. He had grabbed his gun and set off in pursuit, firing at the pigs as he ran. This, in turn, enraged the owner of the pigs, who retaliated by stoning the gunman. The pig man was the better shot, which is why we were called to treat our driver. After admitting him for observation, we stitched up his wound. He did not look too bright (he obviously wasn't), but it was probably his pride which had suffered most. To rub it in still further he would have to attend the police station the next morning and that was at Salelologa, at the other end of the island. Served him right! I had no sympathy for him, particularly as the incident had loaded me with a pile of police forms to be filled in.

Time passed by and June slipped into July. We were now well into the dry season and we were gradually beginning to contemplate our return to 'civilisation'.

The police called in to see me again. They asked me to write a report to be produced in court. It concerned an assault case, not the one involving our driver and the pig farmer, but one which had occurred even before we had arrived on Savaii. They wanted me to state whether the victim of the assault had been struck with a wooden object, or a metal one – and whether it had been blunt or sharp. I had thought that the post-mortem on the non-existent body was the ultimate in absurdity, but this request for a witness statement, when I had never seen the perpetrator, the victim or the weapon, really took the biscuit.

My opinion of Alua has taken another knock. I knew that she was no great shakes as a nurse, but I had rated her very highly as an administrator. Now I discovered that, as a result of a mix-up on the staff rota, which she herself had compiled, she was scheduled to be on duty at the same time as attending a meeting in Apia. As a result, she had simply gone off to the meeting, leaving Maria, a totally incompetent, and totally pregnant, nurse in sole charge of the hospital for three days and three nights. Thank heavens I had Sue. As usual, she would hold the fort.

The Highs and the Lows

Some days later we were pleasantly surprised when Steve and Ava turned up at Sataua. Incidentally, whilst we knew them as Steve and Ava Brown, in Samoa Ava was known by her full name of Lumaava. Her father had been a village chief of high rank and she therefore had the distinguished title of Lumava Funealic Lumaava Sooae Malalag. Sue and I could now understand why she had been a little reluctant to celebrate her wedding on Niue. For someone of her position it would have been unthinkable. Anyway, on this occasion, when they arrived at the hospital, they invited us to lunch at the Vaisala Hotel, which was only about three miles further on around the coast. Unfortunately I had to stay behind to deal with a patient who had just arrived, but Sue went off with them and I promised to join them as soon as I could get away. The new patient had delivered her baby at home, but had not managed to expel the placenta, the afterbirth. It actually delivered quite easily, so all was well and I was able to head off to the hotel. We were just starting to enjoy the barbecue, with an accompaniment of live music, when Soo turned up. She gave me the distressing news that the patient's newly born baby had died. I thanked her for the information but felt that, if the baby were already dead, then there was nothing I would be able to do. We therefore finished our meal before Sue and I hurried back to the hospital. When we arrived, we found that the staff had wrapped the baby up beautifully and put little red flowers on its breast. It was just too emotional for words. Steve and Ava arrived back a little later and stayed the night in our second bedroom.

The following morning was marked by the continuing absence of traffic, with no buses, or vehicles of any kind. Steve told us that everything was at a standstill, even on the main island of Upolu. He explained that this was due to the fact that the gentleman responsible for ordering fuel supplies for the whole of Samoa had gone on holiday. The result was queuing at petrol pumps all over Samoa. However, petrol was the least of our worries. We were more concerned about the lack of drugs. Even paracetamol was now on ration.

We were still trying to find a way to make the local chicken meat soft enough to eat. No wonder the Polynesians had such massive jaws. We mentioned the problem to Steve, who had an instant solution: "Put the meat in a pan with two large lumps of volcanic rock. Cover with water and boil for one hour. Throw away the meat and eat the rocks."

To receive post was such a rare event that it was always a thrill, even if, as on one occasion, it came via the good offices of the Forestry Commission. The package was from Jacky, our New Zealand doctor friend based in Apia. It was a most welcome surprise, a largish box of various antibiotics. I wondered how she had found out about our shortage.

Despite it being the dry season, there were still regular rainstorms and in the second week of July we had one such downpour. It came into and through everything. The slatted windows were a farce, as least as far as keeping out the rain was concerned. Everything was soaked. Sue found a large sheet of polythene in our luggage and, once things had dried out, she used that to cover our clothing and other susceptible possessions. She hoped it would also keep out some of the creepy-crawlies. The rain seemed to come in waves and, when it did, the temperature dropped quite markedly.

The depression at having our belongings soaked was alleviated by the arrival of Luanna, who brought us some fresh bottled water, some fresh fruit and some cheese. Thank heavens for the Svensens. As Sue said, life without them would have been so much harder for us.

Alua was in trouble. She had refused to go to a <u>very important meeting</u> of managers at Palauli hospital. Not only was she the only trained midwife left in the area, but also the only nurse on the duty roster over this period. I heard on the grapevine that she had been disciplined for failing to attend the meeting, but no one said anything to me, or I would have gladly given them my opinion. The usual attitude was, if meetings interfere with nursing, then to hell with the nursing. I applauded Alua's decision, on this occasion, to put nursing first. It was rumoured that she was reprimanded by the Nursing Superintendent Specialist, even though her attendance would have entailed leaving the hospital with no staff. I felt that the only relieving features about this place were my dedicated staff and the beautiful view.

The net result of all this was that Alua was in a very bad mood. She was venting her spleen on all and sundry. If those in authority had half her commitment and consideration for the patients, ... oh, well, what's the use? As Alua herself said to me one day, "The only doctors who seem to care about the Samoans are the *papalagis*."

Other rumours related more specifically to ourselves. It seemed that very favourable reports were being received back at base and this seemed to be upsetting some of those in authority. It would appear that they were happier with the previous Samoan doctor, the one who would apparently stay in bed most of the day, drink himself silly and, as I had just discovered, write out fake prescriptions. Morphia and pethidine, which were supposedly for patients, were used to support his own habit. From what we heard, the authorities were still trying to hush it all up. What was even worse, it seemed that they were trying to throw the blame on one of the junior nurses, as she had actually issued the drugs; the poor girl was just obeying orders from her superior, the Doctor. If she had disobeyed him, then she would have been reported for not carrying out his instructions. It was a classic Catch 22 situation and was also a painful reminder of what had occurred on Tokelau.

Later that week we had an unexpected visit from the forestry people. On this occasion, Ian was accompanied by a Belgian and their driver, a Samoan. We got into conversation and the

Samoan mentioned to Sue that his wife was pregnant. He then asked me if he could bring her to the hospital for me to supervise during the pregnancy. I had no objection, so I agreed. I did not know whether this was the real reason for their visit, but when that bit of business was dealt with, they proceeded to unload their truck. We could hardly believe our eyes as all manner of goodies were carried over to us, Coca-cola, beer, chocolate and fresh vegetables. Wonderful!

They had come from the logging camp, where they were responsible for the machinery. They were rough, hands-on lads, but they struck me as very intelligent. They told us how the trees on the island were being steadily cut down, which had potentially disastrous consequences, with the thin topsoil being easily washed away. They said there was a small team, headed by a young woman from New Zealand, tasked with re-foresting the cut area, but even they admitted that, for every acre cut down, only one square yard was replanted. It was madness. Sweden had an alternative strategy, where they paid the villagers not to let the trees be cut down but instead of investing the aid funds in village facilities and infrastructure, they would just use it to build bigger churches and bigger houses for the priests and other religious leaders. Sometimes the situation on Samoa looked hopeless.

As we sat outside one evening, we listened to the sounds of screaming coming from the hospital ward. The way the Samoans instilled discipline into their children was to beat them unmercifully. They used what looked like a witch's broom and beat them until they had learned absolute obedience and deference to age. It was as though they were taking out all their frustrations on their children. I could understand their frustrations, but their beating of the children I couldn't understand. Eventually Sue couldn't stand it any longer and went to see what was going on. The woman stopped the beating, to see what Sue wanted, Sue just held out her arms towards the child, who ran into them. Sue picked her up and walked off with her, without saying a word. According to Margaret Mead, this sort of family violence just did not occur. SHE WAS SO WRONG ABOUT SO MANY THINGS.

By this time we were getting desperate, not this time for water, or for diesel, or for medical supplies, but for money. We had been promised that we would receive some by now, but nothing had materialised. Our driver had just been around, asking the staff whether they had received their pay. Joe, the paymaster, had not returned from Apia. He had been gone for a very long extended weekend and he should have been back with the pay for everyone. It was now nearly seven weeks since anyone had received any pay from the government. Sue told me that even our resources were stretched to the limit. It was time to ring Terry in Apia and find out what was happening.

Of course, it was not only money, which was 'conspicuous by its absence'. The previous night I had had to wash in a bucket of water, after I had first washed the patient, whose scalp I was about to stitch up; the result of another drunken brawl. Again the lack of water was due to someone emptying the fresh water tanks by doing the family wash. They had then walked away without turning off the taps. We were really fed up; no money, no transport and no water. We decided to do what everyone else did; we would go on holiday. We contacted Manase. They said they would come and pick us up. "Thank you, Terry," and, even more so, "Thank you, Luanna." O.K., so I would be asked to examine a few people and I would have to visit Luanna's family, but that was a small price to pay. Even though we had no cash, we would be allowed unlimited credit at the desk at Manase. What a relief! We would be collected at 8 o'clock on the Saturday morning and brought back late on the Sunday evening. Sue was already packing her bag.

Fortunately she packed for me too. Otherwise I would have arrived with just my Swiss army knife and snorkel!

The weekend went so fast. We met so many people and Sue was very happy. It was like a summer holiday.

All too soon it was over and it was home again, clipperty clop, clipperty clop. And once we got home, it was as if we had never been away. There was still no water, and to make things even worse, the electricity went off in the middle of breakfast. Perhaps they had not paid the bill! Later in the morning I was given a copy of the Samoan Observer, the local paper. The leader purported to explain why the power supply was intermittent. Everyone seemed to know exactly what the reason was, except, that is, for the Samoan authorities. Even we had had it explained to us often enough.

It came back to the deforestation of the island and the gradual removal of the tree cover. When it rained, the soil was just washed away. It washed down the hillsides and into the collecting dams for the hydro-electric power station. This inevitably choked the inlets to the turbines. The designers of the hydro-electric scheme had not anticipated that there would be logging on the hillsides, so no measures had been incorporated to counter the build up of silt.

There was a second factor at work. Our village had voted for the wrong party at the last election. Therefore the promised pumping station had been immediately cancelled. In Samoa it did not pay to vote for the losers. In fact, the village, which had been virtually destroyed by the last hurricane, had received no government assistance with rebuilding. Maybe next time they would think twice before voting for the wrong party!

It was only as we were being shown the damage caused by the hurricane that we realised that there had been a landing strip in the vicinity. Across the bay, joining two spits of beach, were the remains of a concrete airstrip. The construction of the strip had transformed the bay into a closed lagoon. We were told that the South Pacific forces had laid the landing strip during the Second World War and it had remained until destroyed by the hurricane. In its heyday, flying boats had used the lagoon and fighter planes the concrete runway.

More Emergencies – Medical and Otherwise

Whenever transport became available, I took the opportunity to visit the outlying dressing stations. On this particular day, we had just reached Foailalo, which was only about 25 km away but which, on account of the state of our vehicle, had taken us an hour to reach. However, we had only been there a short time, when we received a radio message "Please return immediately. Maternity case. Something very wrong." I had a quick look at the most urgent cases and advised the others that they would have to make their own way to the hospital at Sataua. Then it was back home as quickly as we could.

In the ward I found a lady, who had been in labour for about eight hours, not in the hospital but at her home in the bush. The delivery was making no progress and she was in considerable pain. On examination I found that she was in deep transverse arrest. There was no way that she could deliver naturally and no way that I could manipulate the baby into the correct position. She was going to need a caesarean section. We had neither the instruments nor the equipment to deal with this situation, so would have to get her to the hospital at Palauli. They, at least, had a proper operating theatre and some instruments.

How on earth would we start? We did not even have any suitable transport. It would take three hours for something to come up from Palauli and then take us back again – and that was far too long for the patient's well-being. Eventually we managed to persuade the Vaisala Hotel to lend us their ten-seater vehicle. Alua set up a drip and we managed to manhandle the poor patient onto a mattress in the vehicle. Then off we went, with all lights blazing, the three of us, the patient, Alua and me; Oh, plus the family, extended family, committee members, well-wishers, holiday makers, Uncle Tom Cobbley and all. There was just room for Sue and me to squeeze in front with the driver.

I performed the operation using the most primitive of anaesthetics and there was no real muscle relaxation. The nurse skilfully changed the oxygen cylinder, but unfortunately for one which was completely empty. The surgical instruments, instead of being placed in the surgeon's hand, were simply dropped onto the patient between her legs. I used the old-fashioned vertical incision, and we got the baby out safely, although it looked somewhat battered and indescribably dirty. It was obvious that the theatre nurse had never seen inside a modern western operating theatre, but she had done her best. And at least there had been a full set of instruments available. The baby remained quiet, but it was alive and seemed well enough. The mother had lain quiet and still, while I had performed the operation. She was probably exhausted.

We stopped three times on the journey home, once to buy something to eat at an open food stall and again when we saw our driver's family vehicle. We transferred across to his pick-up, leaving the hotel bus to transport the rest of the company back to Sataua. The final stop was for the simple reason that we ran out of petrol. However, as everyone knew everyone else and they all seemed to be related, it was not too difficult to borrow a jug of fuel. As to the reason we switched vehicles, well it was not entirely to reduce the congestion on the bus. Our driver was only paid for the time he was actually driving and he had not been able to do much of that recently. The hospital vehicle was still incapacitated. In fact, we feared it was in the car mortuary, or wherever cars were taken when they had passed their 'use-by' date. Not that anything was ever wasted. Older vehicles were cannibalised of any useable parts – and the mechanical cannibals even cannibalised the cannibalised vehicles. As our replacement vehicle had, it seemed, been 'acquired' by someone higher up the pecking order in Apia, the outlook, particularly for our poor driver, looked bleak.

When we arrived back home at our hospital, it was to find that Soo had been into our home and had left some food for us. She was very kind and thoughtful. Sue was really tired and went off to bed, but I had to do a ward round. In the main ward, we had a little albino child with her mother. As soon as she saw me, she came running over, as only a child can. Whereas some of the other children were somewhat scared and hesitant concerning *papalagis*, because our colour was different, she had no such caution. We both looked the same, so I was O.K. and I received a great big kiss and a hug. It was these little things, which made it all worthwhile.

Two days later, there was a sense of lightness in the air, a lessening of the tension. The staff had been paid. We too had received some money; not all of it; that would be expecting too much; but we had to be grateful for small mercies. We would at least be able to pay off our small debts, and, in particular, our debts to Manase.

The air was alive with gossip. Something was 'going on' in the government. The local newspaper, The Samoa Observer, ran the headline that 20% of the government income (or was it the country's income?) was being spent to support the state airline, Polynesian Airways. The truth was that there were so many fingers reaching into the pot, that I was surprised there was anything left in the pot, except fingers. The current rumour was that, because the airline's planes did not have the sophisticated electronic equipment to detect approaching aircraft so as to avoid collisions, they would not be allowed to land on any airfields under American control. As one of Polynesian Airways' prime destinations was Eastern (or American) Samoa, this would severely restrict their operations.

The story was being vigorously denied by the government. In fact the newspaper reported that the Prime Minister, Tofilau, had intervened and had spoken with President Clinton himself. Everything was now O.K. and he, the Prime Minister, had a letter from the President giving him the go-ahead. When asked in parliament to produce the letter, he said it was not available 'at this time'.

A further detail of the scandal, as reported in the newspaper, was that Qantas, who were contracted to do the work on the planes, had done nothing and intended to do nothing until the funding was guaranteed by a body acceptable to Qantas.

This business with Polynesian Airways had really shaken the country. The company's finances were so irregular that the directors had arranged for a bill to be passed in parliament to divest them of legal responsibility and to protect them against any claims of impropriety. Not only had the government indemnified the directors against any legal action, but they had backdated the legislation so as to protect even previous board members, who had been replaced in the wake of the disclosure that the airline had accrued a $50 million debt, or so the story went.

Word must have got round that we had received some pay. We were approached by several members of staff requesting to borrow from us, but they had such a lovely way of doing it. "I would like to owe you some money." Good, wasn't it?

That evening we admitted a woman, whose right forearm had been nearly severed. We were told that it had been done by her son! We patched her up and made her comfortable.

At 7 o'clock the next morning we were woken with an urgent message. "Please come across to the theatre now. Urgent!" It was again a case of a complication in childbirth. Her baby had been born, but the woman was bleeding like a stuck pig. Her uterus felt firm, but as I did not have the appropriate instruments to allow me to check inside, I had to go on guesswork. I proceeded to pack the vagina, using at first the correct packing material but, when that was exhausted, being reduced to using sanitary pads. The next stage was to get the patient down to Palauli, where there were more facilities. This time we borrowed a vehicle from Toy Eva. It was pouring down with rain, so we were not thrilled to get two blowouts, the second being about a quarter of a mile from Palauli. The patient was carried the last bit of the way to the hospital. Once in the Palauli operating theatre I felt safe. It was so much better equipped than Sataua. We put up some blood and started to have a look. We removed all the packing and, to my relief, she was as dry as a bone; not a drop of blood to be seen. She would be fine.

Back at the ranch, as the saying goes, Alua had a few surprises for us.

A man had been admitted with a filthy great bandage around his right foot. It was so encrusted with dried blood and dirt, that Alua had been afraid to try to get it off. A lot of warm water soon revealed the painful truth and we listened to the man's story. Several days previously, he had been working up the mountainside, further round the island, cutting small timbers on his plantation, when he had missed the branch and his machete had cut into his foot instead. Unfortunately he had not enough money to get onto the bus, so he had had to wait until his wife could borrow some cash from a relative. (It was only a matter of some small change for the bus fare.)

When I examined the wound, I found that he had virtually amputated his great toe. All I could do was to complete the removal of the remains of the toe and generally tidy up the rest of the foot. I then injected him full of everything I could find in the vaccine cupboard, including antibiotics and tetanus serum. I could be sure that he had never been inoculated against anything. We got him down to the ferry and on to the next boat, on route to the National Hospital at Apia.

After cleaning myself up, I had grabbed a bite of breakfast and was making my way back across to the hospital, when two rather scruffy looking lads turned up carrying surfboards. They claimed to be doctors. They handed me a letter of introduction from Mr. Smith, the Superintendent of the National Hospital in Apia. In a few words, it informed me that the two young men were medical students. I assured them that I would be grateful for any help that they were willing to offer, especially in casualty. I looked forward to them returning from their swim, but that was the last I saw of them. In fact, it was the last anyone saw of them. I suspected that they may have been looking for free board and lodging, rather than actual work experience, or it may have been even less honourable than that. We did not have much of value at the hospital, but nothing was locked away. Anyway, it had been a good try.

An End in Sight

Time marched on and soon it was Tuesday 12th July 1994, which will go down as 'yellow banana day'. Luanna had sent her brother, who had a plantation near to the hospital, to bring us some massive bunches of ripe bananas. Sue was overjoyed. What a feast!

By the Friday, 15th July, we found ourselves glancing at the calendar quite regularly. We were obviously beginning to think about time and to contemplate our return to the 'real world'. On that day we received another gift, not bananas this time, but more drugs from Jacky. We were very grateful. It was just what we needed.

On the Saturday morning, we delivered Ian's wife. Ian insisted that we went off to the Vaisala Hotel to wet the baby's head. In the hotel we met a woman who said that she was selling computers, with a full back up service, or so she claimed. She explained that her next stop was Borneo. If they had the same intermittent electricity supply as we had on Savaii, then it was going to be great fun and a busy time for the 'back up' part of the business.

After showing Warren round with another load of tourists, we went to Iufi's home, where we had been invited for a meal. She also had visitors. They were from Germany and friends or relatives of her husband. The guy was a photographer and he presented us with a signed copy of his book on Samoa. It was very beautiful. I just wished that we were able to take photographs like that. For one thing, we wouldn't waste quite so many films! Incidentally his name was also Max, Max Schwoerer.

I could not quite get a grip on it, but everything seemed to be slowing down. It was like watching a film going slower and slower. Maybe we were finally settling in to the Samoan pace of life.

On the Sunday there was a wedding in the village. The weather was holding, so it was sunny and dry as the couple, in all their finery, walked down the road to the church, followed by a band and a procession of guests and villagers. An hour later they all walked back up the road to their *fale*, with the band playing louder and more enthusiastically than ever.

We had a dinner invitation. It was from a middle-aged Australian couple, on holiday on Savaii. I had treated him the previous week. Whilst out swimming he had compacted the wax in his ear, which necessitated a simple suction clearance to enable him to hear properly again. Still it was nice of them to invite us out to dinner at the Vaisala Hotel, which we were told was owned by one of the government ministers.

A couple of days later, Steve called in to see us. He stayed for lunch and either mistook the time or forgot that he had to leave. Anyway, the outcome was that he missed the ferry and therefore returned for supper and the use of a bed. It was a good job that we had an emergency tin of corned beef. We had a fish starter and then the corned beef with fried breadfruit and tomato. The fridge and the larder were now empty.

Just when we had given up all hope of any assistance, the laboratory in Apia sent over two 'technicians' to sort out our glucose meter, which was an essential piece of equipment if we were to be able to test our diabetic patients. The technicians proved to be worse than useless. They couldn't fix it, so wanted to take it back to Apia. I suspected that, if they did that, it would simply be put on a shelf and forgotten. Anyway, I took out the batteries, as I knew that, if we ever did get a replacement, it would arrive without batteries.

We were now counting the days. It was 21st July, so we had just over a month to go until my work permit expired. I think that the realisation of this prompted us to see as much as we could of Savaii before we left. Therefore when Steve arrived on his motorbike, Sue jumped at the chance to join him on a trip to visit some caves at Papa Beach, about a mile or so around the bay from the hospital. Steve had heard reports that there were rare bats roosting in the caves, but they we unable to find them.

We had again been invited to spend a few days at Manase, so, after the visit to the caves, Steve stayed with us overnight and then took us to Manase on his motorcycle the following day. Actually, it wasn't quite like that. I knew that I would not be able to leave the hospital until the Staff Nurse came on duty in the afternoon, so Steve took Sue and agreed to come back for me later.

By about 3 o'clock in the afternoon, I had done everything that had to be done in the hospital and was ready when he arrived back. With one rucksack on my back and another with the camera equipment on my chest, I sat on the pillion and hung on to Steve for grim death. My feeling of trepidation was heightened by the fact that Steve was holding on to a massive fish that was resting across the handlebars. We were about half way to our destination when Steve pulled off to a small village to deliver the fish. We were not allowed to leave without sampling the local cava, their home brew, which was not only intoxicating and analgesic, but also mildly hallucinogenic. This was followed by a glass of hot chocolate and a lot of chit-chat between Steve and the Elders. While we were there, I examined two men, one of whom had ruptured a muscle carrying a sack of cement half way up a mountainside. Anyway, eventually we got on our way and, bum sore and weary, finally arrived at Manase. What I had not realised until that minute was that the expedition would include more than just Steve, Sue and myself. In fact most of the Hash Harriers were there. They had all driven over from Apia. Only Dr. Jacky and her husband missed the reunion. Their car had had a puncture on the way to the ferry and so had missed the boat. This was a regular occurrence on Samoa. Most of the vehicles had second hand tyres to start with, so it was always a matter of chance as to whether one would finish a journey, however early one set off. Even the little Cessna aircraft had blown a tyre some three weeks previously, and it had not yet been repaired or replaced. The second of the Cessnas was also incapacitated. It had run out of space when it was landing at Apia and had hit something in the grass, spun round and run into the fence. Nothing serious, but there was no repair kit available… but I digress.

As such a large number of the Hash Harriers had arrived for the weekend, we all decided to sleep in the beach *fales*, along the sea front, four or five to a *fale*. It would be much cheaper that way.

Actually it was rather funny. Although we were unaware of it, the choice of this particular date for our stay was a 'set up'. While staying with Steve and Ava, they must have inveigled out of Sue the date of our wedding anniversary. Thus it came about that Steve and Terry had decided that Sunday 24th July was a date to be celebrated. Sue would have been more than happy with a card and a bunch of flowers, but that was not part of the plan. What was produced was an anniversary chocolate cake, beautifully decorated, with the greeting 'Happy 50th Anniversary' emblazoned in bright icing sugar across the top. I glanced over and saw a frown on Sue's face. The intention had been admirable, but as Sue was, at the time, only in her early fifties, the effect was not quite what Steve and Terry had intended. I smiled at Sue and she giggled softly. It was the thought which counted. To make sure the occasion went off with a swing, Terry had arranged a staff band group, who played and danced most beautifully for us. We all had a ball. Sue was up on the little stage, doing her best, dancing with the girls – and she was good. It really was very generous of Terry and Ava to have laid on such a celebration for us. I suppose it was not really *just* for us, as Terry had brought along a lot of other guests, including an MP, whom he insisted that we meet. He had also brought an impressive selection of Australian wines. We had a very liquid night and a wonderful weekend, meeting so many friends and acquaintances. It is the only time we have celebrated our wedding anniversary in the Samoan style, but it is one we shall never forget.

The following morning the younger members of the group, among whom Sue proudly presented herself, went off caving, or tunnelling underground in the lava fields. It must have been exciting, exploring the tunnels in the pitch black, with cave swifts overhead, swooping in and out, carrying food to their nests. The group had a local guide, but he was more scared than they were, not because of the bats, or the crevasses, or the numerous side tunnels, but because of the spirits…!

Sue returned to Manase absolutely exhausted from her climb down the volcanic chimney and she slept like a log, despite the hard floor of the beach *fale*. Her exhaustion could not hide her exhilaration, nor her enthusiasm, for, with little encouragement from Steve, she soon jumped on the back of his motor cycle for a further expedition, again looking for rare bats in another of the cave complexes.

It had been a memorable weekend and it was with great reluctance that, at 4 o'clock on the Monday morning, we clambered into the truck of the lads from the forestry commission, who had offered us a lift back home. We had had a super time, but now it was time for work again.

I returned to find that a small baby had been brought into the hospital. It appeared that someone had tried to circumcise it and, in the process had nearly de-gloved its penis. I did the best I could, but the mother was apparently in Apia and all I could get out of the father was the single word 'Can't'. I wrote a quick note to the National Hospital in Apia and got them off to the ferry. Some time later, while ringing me on some trifling matter, the hospital casually informed me that they had circumcised the baby, as requested! I had that 'Alice in Wonderland' feeling again!

I little thing brightened my day. It was when Alua commented on how steady my hands were when operating. I had not thought about it before. Still it was nice to know how others saw it.

We managed to obtain another copy of the Samoa Observer. It had been publishing confidential reports of correspondence between the government-run Polynesian Airlines and the Public Works Department. It was just as in the western world. The 'secret' government papers had been leaked to the press. According to the reports, there was corruption in the whole system, involving entire families. Of course, that was the *Fa'aSamoa*, the Samoan way, a government minister had a duty to support not only his immediate family, but his extended family as well.

The Observer newspaper was taking a great risk in publishing these articles. Its office had already been burnt down once, because it had printed such uncomplimentary articles.

I was talking with the Reverend Apineru, who was the Methodist minister in the neighbouring village of Asau, which lay just beyond the Vaisala Hotel. He confirmed that the reason that there was no fresh water was, as we had thought, due to politics. The government had been drilling for water, but then came the general election and a referendum on the proposal for V.A.G.T. (value added general tax). Asau had voted against the government, so now no funds would be available for the development of Asau or for our hospital. It was worse than Tammany Hall!

Transport was a continuing problem. It was a case of beg, borrow, or steal. Well, not actually steal, but hire, with a little coercion. Iufi's husband charged us $80 for the use of his vehicle and when we used the vehicle from the Vaisala Hotel then the charge was $200. They told us we were getting it on the cheap, as the usual charge was $300. If the patient had to be taken all the way to Apia then we paid $600.

The following day we were down to three nurses. Alua had gone off to Apia for another meeting, catching the 6.00 a.m. boat. This meant that the nurses had to work anything up to 16-hour shifts. I despaired at this failure to organise properly; it was no better than on Tokelau. In fact, in some ways we found conditions better on Tokelau than here on Savaii. The people had looked after us very well. On Samoa I had to admit that we were often very hungry. I looked back with some fondness to Tokelau and its people.

Samoa and Tokelau had one thing in common, the flexibility of their use of language. 'Immediately' meant 'some time today', and 'see you later' meant 'you may see me tomorrow'.

As I walked across to the hospital, my heart sank. A whole congregation of relatives was just disappearing into our isolation ward. Some of them were even carrying babies and young infants. I despaired. Rightly or wrongly I discharged the patient there and then. At least I could protect our water supply, even if I couldn't protect the patient. They could do their weekly wash back at home.

Two days later Alua arrived back from her conference. She brought us $20 worth of stuff from the market, but then presented us with a bill for $40. It served us right. We had been caught out like this before. Would we never learn? We always expected the best and were always disappointed. Alua arrived back just as we had admitted a two-week-old baby with an abscess on its left breast the size of a golf ball. The baby was so dirty; I had seen pigs which were cleaner.

After that a patient arrived with a sore ear. The Samoans seemed to have a predilection for putting things into any bodily orifices they could fine. This one had stuffed something into his ear. Then he had tried to get it out by ramming even more stuff in. What a mess! I managed to clear the ear canal with a fine water jet made from a rusty spinal injection needle. I could then at least see what I was looking at. He had ruptured his eardrum. All I could do was to remove the muck and gubbins using a fine suction tube and to clean it up. I packed the ear, gave him some antibiotics and sent him across to Apia.

By the time I had finished, it was seven in the evening and I was just packing up when I heard the mysterious horn blower. I also noticed that the hospital's fresh water supply had been turned off. My mass ejection of the relatives had been for nothing.

We reached 31st July and I was feeling relatively fresh. I had only been called out once during the night. This was to show the nurse how to relieve the pain of a bleed underneath a fingernail. By drilling a fine hole into the nail, or at least, by heating up a needle and burning a fine hole through the nail, I was able to let the locked up blood escape. I suppose it's easy when you know how.

Warren had not been around for a couple of weeks and I was down to the last book from his 'library'. It was 'Family and Kinship in East London'. It was a Pelican book and a very good read, being a socially uplifting treatise written at the beginning of the twentieth century by the Fabian Society and describing social conditions at that time. There were considerable parallels with what we had experienced in the South Pacific.

Sue and I had both noticed that we had begun to put weight back on again. Maybe the invitations to lunch at the hotel and the weekend with the Hash Harriers had had something to do with it. It had been good to be slim, or, at least, slimmer, but not quite so good to be hungry!

Our next emergency was an ectopic pregnancy. The patient's blood pressure had dropped to the floor and the nurse had spent about an hour looking for a blood donor. She had not realised that Sue was a 'universal donor', whose blood was compatible with all blood groups. I quickly stabilised her condition, but we had no equipment in Sataua for this sort of case. It was essential to get her off to Apia quickly. 'Quickly' in this case meant waiting over an hour for the ambulance to arrive from Palauli. Sometimes one had to appreciate the service we had back home in England. Although the ambulance was only equipped to carry one patient, it had to make room for the entire family, plus cooking utensils, and, last but not least, a committee member. She was there, she said, to see fair play, whatever that might mean.

That afternoon I received my first and only lesson in native pharmacology. From the two young men in the public health team, I learned that the way to treat hepatitis was as follows:

Scrape off the bark of Lychee, Wild Croton, Pometa pinnata and Variegatrum moluccanum, discarding the dead outer skin.

Mix equal amounts of these ingredients with water. Kneed the mixture and filter.

Drink for four days to effect a cure.

It certainly sounded interesting, especially as they insisted that it was also very good for toxoplasmosis. Sue and I preferred to put our faith in not drinking the local water. I consumed a colossal number of coconuts for their juice and Sue went through crates of Coca-Cola, whenever she could get it. Not that we had much choice that day. The water was off again, so there was none either for drinking or for making exotic medicines.

The weather had turned and, although it was still warm, the wind was beginning to howl. This meant that there was very little fishing done and we had some difficulty in finding some fish to buy for our meal.

The following day, I received another lesson in the local language. We were visited by a young woman who had had her ovaries removed. Her medical records did not give the reason. Anyway, her question was: would she still be able to have 'Oos', and how many Oos could he make for her before he had an Ahh? I have reproduced it as accurately as I can, and as honestly as I am able; I was learning.

What I never learned or understood were the thought processes of local officialdom. After having suffered from a lack of water for several days, we discovered that the Donkey, the name that J.C. had given to our Health Inspector, had turned off the main stop cock under a grating, but had then forgotten to inform anyone. Before he had left us, J.C., by way of a little chit-chat, had told me that several of the Savaii villages had had their water pumps removed for not paying their bills. This made me wonder whether there could be any connection between this and the high incidence of typhoid around Palauli and Faleolupo. Perhaps they were being forced to use the water from the local streams.

We wondered why there had been a sudden fall off in the number of maternity cases coming to the hospital. Then we found out that the Committee had issued an edict that each patient had to bring with them two packets of sanitary pads. Most of the patients just could not afford them, so we were only seeing those cases which were too complicated for the local midwife, or 'handy woman'. Sue immediately went on the warpath and shot off in search of the Committee. They had better beware. I decided to keep out of the way on this one.

After having an afternoon cup of tea, I went across to see that everything was all right in the hospital. It was a good job I did. Alua had screwed up again. For someone who seemed to be a sound administrator, she was making a surprising number of mistakes. This time she had given nurse Maria time off and not remembered to inform anyone. Over the same period I had given Iufi time off because, as from the following Monday, both she and 'Number Nine' would have to work flat out through the whole week. It would be inoculation time for the schoolchildren. As a result I found Soo, our loyal Nurse Aid, not only working alone, but expected to work three days and nights without respite. When I arrived she was struggling with a blocked drip.

As I was sorting out that little problem, I noticed some excitement outside the hospital. A vehicle had just knocked down a young child. The driver was apparently intending to drive on, but some of the villagers saw the incident and forced him to stop. (It was quite usual for a vehicle not to stop after an accident.) It was a government vehicle, carrying a group of Japanese. There was not a glimmer of expression or concern on the face of any one of them. The child was fortunately not seriously injured and the driver soft soaped its father. He was, after all, a government driver and this a government vehicle, and the child was only bruised.

It was Sunday and we had to really rack our brains as to what to have for Sunday dinner. We had nothing substantial in the larder, so it had to be Sunday mish-mash. This consisted of yam and onion mashed up with a hard boiled egg and seasoned with salt, pepper and some old ketchup. To this was added the finely chopped remains of a hoarded piece of cabbage and some even more treasured pieces of cucumber and carrot. All this was then mixed together with some out-of-date mayonnaise. It tasted surprisingly… well, yes, surprisingly!

To finish the meal off, Soo brought in a bowl of spaghetti and turkey tails. The spaghetti was all right, although a bit salty. As for the tails, well, a little dog, which had adopted us, must have thought it was his birthday! As if our meal had not depressed us sufficiently, we looked out of the window and saw that it was just like a wet and dismal afternoon at Filey. If you don't know where Filey is, or what it looks like on a wet and dismal day in summer, then I can tell you that it is about as dispiriting as mish-mash mayonnaise!

It was early Monday morning 15th August 1994 and a number of vehicles had pulled up at the hospital to collect our nurses. It was time to start the inoculation of the local schoolchildren. For our nurses it would be a week of hard labour and Sue had been asked to go with them. She would no doubt find plenty of anecdotes to record in her private journal.

All went well for the first day, but on the second morning, the driver of one of the vehicles found that he had insufficient petrol to complete the day's programme. The driver had neither the money nor a government purchase chit to purchase fuel from the petrol station just a stone's throw down the road from the hospital. He advised us that he would have to go back to Palauli in a vehicle which he had stopped and persuaded to undertake the trip, in order to get some petrol from the Administrator, a round trip of about three hours. In the meantime, the schools would have to remain closed. I decide to keep out of it.

A couple of the nurses took the initiative upon themselves and persuaded another driver to take them in his car to a nearby school, so that they could do some work. For this they had offered to pay him two dollars. I was lost for words. Perhaps it was no bad thing that there was only one more week before my work permit expired!

After observing what was happening both on Tokelau and in Samoa, we had had to conclude that, however much it had distressed us, the underlying picture was very much the same as in the west. It was just that the west was very much more sophisticated in the way it operated. We may not recognise this, as we always tended to judge others by our own standards, without taking account of their different customs and fashions. We had often been very frustrated by the lifestyle and attitudes of the people of the South Pacific, but no more so than we were by the intervention of the Christian Aid Workers. As Sue had said to me as they were leaving, "These boat do-gooders are really just earning themselves a few extra Brownie points on their way up to Heaven." We all had our own personal agendas.

On 18th August (now we really were counting the days), we admitted a patient who had been involved in a hit and run accident. He had sustained a closed chest injury. With no X-ray equipment, there was nothing we could do for him, so again it was a case of 'make him as comfortable as possible and ship him off to Apia'.

Our next patient had received a machete wound during the night. When he reached us in the morning, he was still covered in pig muck. As usual the normal medical ethic of thoroughly washing one's hands had to be strictly observed, but this was the first time where I had felt it even more necessary to scrub up *after* dealing with the patient than before going in to treat him! I made damned sure that I scrubbed my hands very carefully after I had finished with that 'unsavoury' character. I had Soo to help me. After I had carefully cleaned the wound, she helped wipe everything with a dirty breech cloth.

The ambulance finally arrived from Palauli, but their new oxygen cylinder would not fit the connection mount. They only had one and a half hours to get to the wharf before the boat left and, as the 'hit and run' patient was looking decidedly the worse for wear, despite the two drips we had fitted up, I asked Alua to radio the boat to ensure that it didn't leave before the patient arrived.

The police contacted us to say that the driver of the vehicle had given himself up. He claimed that he had driven off to save himself from the anger of the villagers. He had driven to the police station in the next village of Asau for safety.

A couple of days later, Warren called in with more news of Polynesian Airways. He said it was really affecting the economy; business was very flat. The airline was no longer flying to a schedule. They had purchased a second hand plane from Kuwait Airlines, but it did not have proximity warning gear fitted. It had therefore been sent to New Zealand to have this omission rectified. Polynesian Airways were no longer operating on any long haul routes and all the passengers who had been booked with them were now 'screwed up'.

So, as we reached the end of this twentieth day of the eighth month, the electricity went off again – and it was only 6 o'clock!

Over the next few days we had a sudden rush of clients, many having small, deep, filthy wounds on their bodies and some of them several days old. The usual cause was stone throwing. Outbreaks of minor violence like this were almost routine. The Samoans could be very quick to take offence, particularly if their status in the local hierarchy were derided, or their self-esteem damaged. I bathed the wounds with peroxide and covered them with ointment from an out-of-date capsule of Chloromycetin (an antibiotic). It seemed to work, or maybe I was just lucky.

Our most dramatic admission was a patient brought to us from the church, where he had collapsed. We were told that he had had diarrhoea for the previous 24 hours and had not eaten or drunk anything. The poor fellow had just fallen forward and given his forehead a good crack on the pew in front of him. We measured his blood sugar – one of the few things we were still able to measure, and tested his urine with our remaining test strips. Good-oh, he was a diabetic. At least we knew how to treat that, and he surfaced quite rapidly after we had got some fluid and some sugar into him.

I was gradually becoming more dispirited. In the absence of Alua, standards seemed to drop quite markedly. It did not help that we had no electricity and the water supply was intermittent, but, as I walked through the hospital, I noticed that everything was dirty; the instrument tray had not been cleaned since I had used it on the previous day and nothing had been sterilised. To make things worse, I was told that a hypertensive patient had been admitted during the night. I felt very uncomfortable at having seriously ill patients in a dirty hospital.

The following Monday morning brought the usual stampede, and the usual administrative chaos. The staff would take the patient's name and then try to find his records. Unfortunately there was no guarantee that the patient was using the same name as on any previous visits; they seemed to change them at will – and he may well have forgotten the name under which he had registered on the last occasion. While the staff were trying to sort this out, the patient would wander off to have a chat with someone in the wards. By the time the case reached me in my room, it would be extremely doubtful if the records I was given bore any connection with the patient in front of me. They may have related to a relative, or simply to someone with a vaguely similar name. On occasions I was even handed a blank sheet of paper; at least I could rely on that to be accurate! The whole system was characteristic of the *Fa'aSamoa*, the Samoan way. In a way, it didn't matter, I still had to patch up the patients, whatever their names. I therefore got stuck in, and cut and stitched all morning. Maybe I was feeling particularly cynical, but I found it difficult to dismiss the thought that the biggest disaster in the South Pacific was its people.

That afternoon marked a significant event, the return of the hospital car. It had been re-sprayed and re-upholstered, and had received five 'new' tyres. In fact it was perfect; well, nearly perfect. I did notice that the four wheels were only held on by eight wheel nuts, which was a shortfall of 60% on the ideal number, and that the hand brake lever was no longer connected to the brakes. It also became apparent very quickly that there was a short circuit somewhere in the electrics, so that the battery had to be disconnected after every journey, to avoid it going flat. As I say, the car was virtually perfect!

Another 'red letter day'. It was 23rd August, which marked the end of my work permit. The day went like a dream and everything went smoothly. The drips works; needles went into veins without any resistance, and the patients had their own names and were generally where I expected them to be. For once I returned to the maternity unit, which had been our home since we had arrived, with a smile on my face.

Of course, the fact that my work permit had now expired meant nothing. No one expected me to 'down tools' and leave. It was just a bureaucratic aberration, like any other in Samoa. I was not due to leave Savaii for another two weeks and I, like everyone else, knew that I would keep working until the last day. However, there was no reason why we should not do something to mark the occasion and so, when I returned to our quarters after my day in the hospital, Sue had prepared a special supper to celebrate. How she had done it, I never knew, but we had lamb chops with potatoes, accompanied by a sauce made with a can of tomatoes, herbs and spices. This was followed by a fruit salad, obtained from the Chinese store.

The meal was a total success, except for the fruit salad, which was 'off'. But then, the tin had been well past its sell-by date. Before complaining to the store, Sue had a look at the other items in our meagre store cupboard. A packet of cheese was a year past its sell-by date. The store gave Sue her money back. No quibble. After the meal we sat listening to excerpts from the Messiah on our old cassette recorder, now back in working order thanks to J.C. Sue had always loved 'The Planets'. The tape was by now almost worn out, but we thought it was bliss.

We sat in the lounge fantasising about what we would like as our first meal when we got back home to Yorkshire; something sweet and sour to start with, then individual Beef Wellingtons, fresh fruit salad, followed by a cheese board, all accompanied by an assortment of good wines.

Before retiring for the night, I went outside to gaze at the stars and to say goodnight to Tapoo. According to Samoan tradition, Tapoo and Tair are brother and sister stars, Tapoo being the night and time to eat, and Tair being the morning and time to get up.

Later in the week we received another message from Warren. Polynesian Airlines were in really deep trouble. We all knew of the stories about the way they had been managed and that some politicians believed that they existed to suit their private convenience. There was the story of the time when a scheduled international flight had been cancelled because the plane had been commandeered to transport the Samoan rugby team and its supporters to Fiji. Of course, it had been a very important match! The scheduled passengers had been stranded and had missed their connections. Never mind. Write it down as an 'Act of God'.

What worried us was that we were also scheduled to fly out with Polynesian. Sue therefore spent considerable time on the radio-telephone, trying to sort it out. This was not easy, as it entailed contacting the National Hospital in Apia so that they could phone the airline and ask them to ring us. We learned that all flights had been rescheduled, but as for assurances…..!

We were honoured to receive a visit from Dr. Bolinson. He kindly wined and dined us at the local hotel. In his own bibulous manner, he related how he had obtained his post as W.H.O. representative. He told me that he was a genuine Doctor, but a Doctor of Geology. During a period when his career was not going too well, his mother had happened to read a job advertisement requiring a Doctor for the World Health Organisation. She thought "Well, my son's a Doctor," so she sent off for an application form. He knew he had no chance, but, to humour her, he filled it in – and got the job.

It was a good evening. I told him about the out-of-date drugs, but he said he already knew all about them. Not only that, but the W.H.O. also knew about the matter. It was, he said, the fault of people on committees, who had friends on other committees. In other words, it was another case of rampant corruption. As usual, it was the local people, the poor and the sick, who suffered for the sins of their representatives.

One of our drivers came into my office to ask if he could borrow the hospital vehicle. He had arranged with one of the nurses, Maria, the very pregnant one, to exchange homes. She lived a fair way off, up on the mountainside, whereas he lived just across the road from the hospital. It was a simple matter of moving pots, pans, sleeping mats and a paraffin burner cooker; oh, and, of course, the children. They owned nothing else. He left at 6 o'clock in the morning, but was back to do his normal day's work.

I had to work the weekend; what a chore! Well, not exactly. I worked it at Svensen's place at Manase. It was another wonderful weekend away, even if we did bring back a patient with us. While we were there, we learned from Adrienne that she was about to leave Savaii. She and her partner had invested in a new enterprise, a guesthouse back on the mainland. Malu was already there, getting it established, while Adrianne completed the process of training up new kitchen staff to replace them at Manase.

We hadn't seen Alua for a week, but now she was back from her various meetings.

That was a relief, as Sue and I had been covering for the shortage of nurses. Apart from Iufi, who was a trained nurse, I had been the only qualified medical cover between Sataua on the western tip of Savaii, and Apia on the north coast of Upolu.

We had one patient who required a blood transfusion. Sitting next to him in the hospital was a relative with the same blood group. Would he give blood to save his kinsman's life? Oh, no. He claimed that he had given blood one month previously. In this situation, Sue felt no compunction to volunteer, so Iufi went off to the village, or rather to the patient's own village. She took with her the blood group bank book and, in her Germano-Samoan accent said "I bring." Sure enough, she did.

Later in the day, Warren arrived with a group of Australian tourists. He made us sound like something out of one of Somerset Maugham's books. We felt flattered, particularly when they offered Sue some chocolates and some packets of Smarties. Talk about a child with a bag of sweeties; she was in her element!

We had managed to buy some frozen chicken (the edible variety) and so that evening we had chicken stew with pawpaw, breadfruit and taro. On this occasion we also had one special ingredient, carrot, with the compliments of Mrs. Luanna Svensen. Who would ever have dreamed that a carrot would be seen as a luxury? Afterwards we relaxed with Dvorak, Tchaikovsky and Bruch. The cassette player and the tapes were, like us, just about on their last legs, but they had seen us through some stressful times and would no doubt last out the final couple of weeks.

We got to pondering; what would we do for Christmas? Sue said that we would just stay at home and have a special roast, in which one bird is de-boned and stuffed with another smaller bird. This in turn is filled with honey and clove ham. It is a recipe, which Sue cooks to perfection. We would accompany it with some good wine. After so many months of virtual abstinence, I craved a good wine!

We would stay at home for Christmas, just Sue and me, and anyone who wished to join us.

At 6 o'clock the next morning, the power went off again. When I went across to the hospital, I had a row with the nurses. They would not get it into their heads that they had to hand over to the incoming nurses before going off-duty. Even if they only gave a verbal report on the patients' health, it would be something. Not that they were unaware of the requirement; I knew that, when Alua was present, she would always insist on it. But when the cat's away.....

Another problem was that of timekeeping. The concept of 'flexi-time', was very natural to the Samoan way of life, but, unfortunately, only as regards coming on duty. When it came to knocking off time, then they observed it to the minute.

Likewise, if we did anything to upset the Committee, then they jumped like mad, but when they were reminded that they had forgotten to provide any food for the nurses on the previous day, they just shrugged.

Sue continued to provide food for the patient whom we had brought back from Manase. She had no relatives at this end of the island, and the Samoan ethic of 'What's mine is yours' did not extend outside their own village.

Custom and tradition were so important, but Sue and I sometimes found them very difficult to come to terms with. There was the case of a young man, a relative of one of the patients, who approached us as we were sitting on a trolley in the hospital, talking to Toy Eva. Crouching very low, he said, "The drip, she stop." Then he backed away, still genuflecting. "What the devil was that all about?" I asked Toy Eva. Oh, she said, it was a mark of respect. Well it may be so, but I didn't like it. As far as I was concerned, human beings stood upright and only animals crouched down. Toy said no, it was just a mark of respect.

Later in the day, a dead body was brought in to our casualty area, followed by a group of wailing females. This grieving choir seemed to be comprised of two groups. As one group reached a particular high note, so the other group took over the screeching. Gradually the wailing became wilder and wilder, with the daughter of the deceased becoming more and more worked up until she lost all control of herself. By this time the room was full of people, all becoming more agitated by the minute. The grieving daughter was by now flailing her arms and throwing herself about. The whole spectacle was in danger of getting out of hand, so, asking Alua for a syringe and an ampoule of tranquilliser, I just approached from behind and, stabbing straight through her clothes I emptied the syringe into her ample rear end.

Soon peace had been restored and I could take stock of the situation. I was at a loss to know what they really wanted. The woman was obviously dead, and had been so for some time. Eventually one of the sons of the deceased explained that he wished to take the body over to the mainland, where his father lived. Somewhere; he was not sure exactly where; he had been gone for some time. In the meantime he wanted us to store his mother's body where we had 'cold'. I pointed out that we had neither mortuary nor cold room and could not possibly store the body. By now it was getting pretty warm, both inside and outside, and already half of the village had gathered to watch the show. All the best vantage points were already taken.

Then the son asked me to instruct the nurses to lay out the body. That was where I drew the line. I pointed out that the woman was already dead when brought into the hospital and it was not the duty of my nurses to act as morticians or funeral directors. It was their responsibility, as the family of the deceased, to perform this last mark of respect. They all knew this; it was just a try-on. I may have been a *papalagi*, but I was not that gullible.

At last the crowd quietened down; the villagers returned to their homes and peace was restored. One of the relatives returned with a new set of clothes for the deceased and the *Matai* (the village family head) arrived to supervise the removal of the corpse. Actually, our main hospital at Palauli had a key to the mortuary at Salelologa, but as I knew that they never manned the radio-telephone in the evening, I decided not to get involved. The *Matai* would have to sort it out.

The following week we went down to Palauli for the regular clinic and, as we had some spare time and petrol, we drove the additional 10 miles around the coast to Safua to see Warren. He was feeling quite pleased with himself. He had been on the Australian television, and the following day he intended to take Sue and me off to see the only woman on the island who still knew how to make *Tapa* or *Tapa au*. This is a material made from the fibrous lining of the bark of the mulberry tree and now only used for ceremonial clothing. It was a very interesting visit and Sue made a good recording of the whole process of making the cloth. It was fascinating, and Warren gave us a running commentary of the whole process starting from where the bark was stripped from a branch of the tree.

Warren also included us in a tour group visit to see the Alofaaga Blowholes, on the south coast of Savaii, about midway between Palauli and our base at Sataua. On the journey, Warren pointed out the large number of dead trees on the sides of the road. They had all suffered from the amount of salt blown on to them during the last hurricane. The subsequent rains had been insufficient to wash the salt off, so very many had perished.

The blowholes performed magnificently, and Warren got some of the locals to throw coconuts into the holes in the periods of calm between spouts. If they got the timing just right, then the coconuts would be blown up to 100 feet in the air. It was quite spectacular. The phenomenon was caused by the sea rushing into the bottom of laval tubes, which were constricted by the partial collapse of the tube sides. The air was therefore compressed as it was forced through the tube, causing a magnificent spray to burst up into the air

On this particular trip there were a number of Australian tourists. They thought that their trip had been very good and that Warren was a superb tour guide. However, their general impression was that Samoa, and everything to do with it, was grossly overpriced, a message they felt they would have to pass on to others back home. Even the one English lad agreed completely with them, as reluctantly did we. We felt that, unless they did something to change the practice of charging five star prices for two star facilities, the Samoans would destroy their own tourist trade.

We later received a message from Steve, who was still waiting for his own tour bus to be completed. He had bought a chassis cab, and the bodywork was being made to his own particular specification. He was very worried at the feedback from Warren's group and feared that this negative reaction from visitors might impact his own fledgling business. He wanted to know what we thought.

Back at Sataua, life went on as usual in the hospital. That is to say, I was again woken just after midnight to attend to an emergency in the labour ward. They could at least have let me sleep another couple of hours, as it was 3.00 a.m. before she finally delivered the baby. It was a baby girl, which was rather unusual. I think it was only the third female baby I had delivered; nearly all of them had been males. As male children were so much more highly valued than girls, this statistic can only have enhanced my reputation.

Eventually we reached the occasion of our last scheduled visit to the hospital at Palauli. It was odd how our arrival on Savaii had coincided with the disappearance of the two doctors who were supposed to be manning that hospital. I suppose I took some pride in having managed to support both hospitals, and the dressing stations, without outside help, but it would have been interesting to know what had happened to them. The gratitude of the staff at Palauli was evidenced by the flower *lei*, which was put around my neck to say 'Thank you'. We would have been rather more appreciative of a bite to eat, as we had eaten nothing since leaving home early in the morning and it was three o'clock in the afternoon by the time we left the hospital.

I arrived back to find a request for a death certificate. It was for the child who had been killed in the road traffic accident the week before. As it had been buried for a week, it was a little late to be considering a post-mortem, but I completed the paperwork, just to keep the bureaucrats happy.

Of rather more concern were several recent incidences of paraquat poisonings and shootings, most of which I doubted were accidental. And Margaret Mead had maintained, despite all the evidence, that the Samoans were a peaceful people.

On 30th August I received a letter officially informing me that I was to finish work on 9th September 1994. I hoped that this letter, together with my work permit (despite it showing an expiry date of 23rd August) would help get us out of the country without too much trouble or expense. This may seem a very odd comment, but it was amazing how many officials would find it essential to see, touch, lose, or misplace these various pieces of documentation and each would insist on applying his own rubber stamp, for which service a demand for money was obviously quite appropriate. We determined that, as soon as we reached Apia, we would obtain a number of photo-copies of each document to ensure that, when we reached the final exit gate, we were still able to prove that we were 'legal emigrants'!

Back in the hospital I was humming as I worked, when one of the nurses complimented me on the neatness of my stitchery. This raised my spirits even more. Maybe I should consider taking up embroidery when we got home; with Sue possibly taking a course in pottery. She had become such a dab hand with the plaster of Paris. Perhaps we could set her up and advertise her abilities, based upon her experience as a bespoke maker of splints to the Sataua hospital. When I suggested this to Sue, she soon put a dampener on it, by pointing out that my greatest expertise lay in the way I could, in any circumstances, manage to get stains on my shirt. Even though, before any work in the delivery room, or any surgical intervention, I would carefully take my shirt off and hang it at the other end of the room, it would still get spattered with blood. The previous day, having donned an apron before starting work, I still succeeded in staining my trousers. Sue stated her opinion that I was just a naturally messy male – and this of a man whose surgical needlework was already becoming legendary!

We had to collect our mail from the shop in the village and, although we enquired every day, the answer was usually "No; no mail!" However, it would be no surprise if, later in the day, someone from the village would come up with a letter for us. There was no telling how long it may have been there, possibly weeks. On one particular day, we were just musing on the fact that in just over a week we would be leaving Savaii, when a letter arrived from Barbara, an old school friend of Sue, living in the South of England. We had written and asked her about making a hotel reservation in London for when we got back. We only wanted to rent a room, not buy the hotel! Christ, the daily cost of the room was equal to what I was being paid for working day and night for four weeks. We had thought how wonderful it would be to get into a comfortable bed, have a good hot bath and a slap-up meal; even the luxury of flicking a switch and having a light come on, without wondering if it would overload the generator, but now it looked as if all that would have to wait until we got home to Yorkshire. If we found that we could afford a brief stay in London, then we would like to take in a show, as we had really missed the cultural life of the west.

With just a week to go, we began to think about our actual departure. Sue refused to contemplate the 6 o'clock ferry, which would have meant getting up at about 3.00 a.m. She insisted we take the 10 o'clock ferry, as suggested by our driver. To be on the safe side, I checked with Toy Eva, whose husband was a ferry captain. It was a good job that I did. There was no 10 o'clock boat.

That morning we had an emergency involving our enlisted nurse, Peony. She had apparently tried to induce an abortion. We rushed her on to the operating table and managed to stabilise her condition. While this was going on, her husband was just wandering around the hospital asking for beer.

As I was cleaning up after the operation, the nurse on duty informed me that she had to go home to get some food. When I asked for an explanation she told me that the Director of Nursing had ruled that the Committee should no longer provide meals for the nursing staff. Apparently the village was split and it depended on where the nurses lived in the village as to whether they would get fed. It was politics again.

In the evening we popped out to the Vaisala Hotel to see their Big Night Floor Show. Sue caught some of it on video, but we did not think it was as good as the impromptu show that the girls at Manase had put on.

Fame at last! I received a message from Dr. Bolinson that the plan, which I had drawn up for rationalising and improving the Tokelauan medical services, was to be presented as the proposal for the country's future. However, as the proposal would be presented by the Director of Medical Services as *his* plan, any credit reflected on me would be ephemeral, if not illusory. Nevertheless I took comfort from the thought that some good might come from our stay in Tokelau.

It was sometimes difficult to know what impact we were having on the local people, but I did notice how, if I did my evening rounds without Sue, both the nurses and the patients would invariably ask, "Where Suzie?" It was clear that she was appreciated as a significant contributor to the teamwork, which we had tried to encourage. Old Soo continued to look upon Sue as her particular responsibility.

I called back to see how Peony was progressing. Her husband, one of our health inspectors was now nowhere to be found. I suspected that he had 'done a runner'.

My conversation with Peony was interrupted by another call to the labour ward. Delivery was being prevented because the baby had the cord around his neck. I was able to free it easily and the birth continued without complication. As may have been anticipated, the baby was christened Max.

I heard Sue muttering about 'messy males' and realised that I had again managed to spatter my clothes. It seemed unavoidable, however high I pulled up my apron.

Thanks to another of the good deeds performed by J.C. during his short visit, our heated baby-bed was now working again. We still had no oxygen feed, but then, one couldn't ask for everything.

We did nearly have one bit of luck. Apparently someone had left a washing machine and a refrigerator to the hospital. They had been delivered, so it was clear that they did actually exist, but somehow they had taken wing during the night and the following day were nowhere to be found. Alua suspected that the relatives of our nurse, Maria, had something to do with it.

By Tuesday 7th September, we realised that we now had very little time left. If we wanted a photographic record of Savaii and its people, then we had to get a move on.

On that day, yet another Max was born. The way things were going they would soon have to change the name of the country from Sam-oa to Max-oa.

We also had an asthmatic patient not responding to treatment. The nurses had failed to identify that it was a case of Cardiac Asthma, rather than the more usual Bronchial Asthma, even though the two are easily distinguishable.

During our final weekend, we went for a walk along the coastal path around our peninsular. At one spot we could see a banana tree growing out of the cliff face and bearing three large bunches of green bananas. Close by there was also a pawpaw tree with fruit. The spot was almost inaccessible, but we would have to try to find someone prepared to climb down and retrieve the fruit. Although we still had a little carrot, onion and potato to go with the last of our frozen chicken, a green banana would enhance it very nicely. We had given up on the native chicken. The meat was so tough and stringy, that even the dog ate it only under protest.

Ian and his family called in to say goodbye to us. On their way out, they were stopped by a member of the local committee, who wanted to charge them for their consultation! What a country!

Payment of our small allowance was again overdue, so we waited in anticipation for our driver to return from Palauli, where Joe, the local paymaster and medical services 'fixer', passed his time. He would never pay the full amount that was due, but always managed to come up with an excuse. The real reason was that the government simply had insufficient money in the kitty, and what little there was had to grease too many palms.

When the driver did arrive, it was not to bring the staff's pay, but to ask me to look at his young son. I could see that the child had pleurisy and I wanted to admit him, but the mother would not let her child stay. All I could do was to give him a much stronger antibiotic than would be usual, as I knew that there was a great likelihood the child would not be brought back for ongoing care. If he didn't return, I would try to find him myself the next morning.

While I was busy treating his son, the driver told me that the hospital previously had its own generator, but it had developed a fault and had been sent to Apia for repair at the beginning of the year. It had never come back. It had been the same story with the X-ray machine.

After almost a year of living in the South Pacific, I was coming to the conclusion that the work ethic was not something which was valued. Those who were most highly respected appeared to be those who did the least work. Our experiences with Mr. Balani, Dr. Liutta and the E.O., not to mention the medical authorities responsible for Savaii, had all convinced us of this.

That is not to say that all the people in positions of authority fell into this category. One exception was the new member of parliament for our district, who had recently visited the hospital. He introduced himself to me as Fritz and, after we had discussed the problems we faced, particularly those caused by the lack of equipment, he asked me if I would be able to provide him with a list of all the things which had gone missing, or had been returned to Apia for repair, etc. I assured him that I would do my best, although much of the information would have to come from the other members of staff, as most of the items had already disappeared by the time I had arrived. He seemed genuinely concerned at what had occurred and told me that most of the missing equipment had been donated by the Japanese government.

Fritz then asked me to accept his personal thanks for the work we had done and offered Sue and me free lodging at his hotel when we returned to Apia. I acknowledged his offer most gratefully. We had already made arrangements for the two days we would spend in Apia before our flight home, but in Samoa one could never be sure …! We knew that Steve and Ava would be as generous as ever, but we also knew that we needed a few days to recuperate. Rest and relaxation were never on the agenda when Steve was around, so we had arranged to stay at a guesthouse for those couple of days. If, for any reason, our departure were delayed, it would be very convenient to take advantage of Fritz's kind offer. As we learned, he was a wealthy businessman, who had spent most of his career in American Samoa, but had been enticed back to Western Samoa to become a member of parliament. He not only owned the Inseln Fehmarn Hotel in Apia, but also had a considerable stake in the Vaisala Hotel on Savaii.

As I had suspected, the driver's child was not brought back into the hospital. I was pleased that I had given it the long acting antibiotic. It never ceased to surprise me how the locals seemed to be dismissive of their children's well-being. It was almost as if their philosophy was 'after all, babies are easy to make'. It was as casual as that.

One of the patients brought Sue a gift, a beautiful little bag and two 18" decorative squares, all hand-made out of the leaf of a *pandanus* palm. On a little label was written 'From Falima and grandchildren'. We have them sitting on our dressing table to this day.

Exactly as on Tokelau, it looked as if there would be a great influx of patients just as we were preparing to leave, a grandstand finale, if you like. I had just completed the amputation of a finger, when we received a call telling us to expect a baby with meningitis, who was being sent over from the other side of Savaii. The radio-telephone was going mad. Now there was a case of pneumonia down at Palauli. When the baby arrived, I found that it had severe bronchiolitis, rather than meningitis, but because of the incorrect diagnosis, it had been given a very large and unnecessary dose of valium, a tranquilliser. Somehow we had to improvise an oxygen tent. It was, and looked, a very makeshift affair, but it worked. We were lucky and, when the parents turned and said "Thank you, Doctor," we were also very happy.

Finally we were ready. Sue had been washing and packing like mad. We had been 'travelling light', so where had all the stuff come from?

Our last evening was very emotional. Many prayers were offered up for us and many presents gratefully received, including one large *letoga-fala-lili-i* (a fine large sleeping mat). I responded as best I could. It was, as I said, very emotional. As I climbed into bed, I determined to get up early to take one last video of the old boat builder at work on a new tree trunk. I had been intending to do it for weeks and this would be my last chance.

On a Wing and a Prayer

The journey back to Upolu, the main island, was as exciting as ever, with the same leaking bow doors. However it was, thank heavens, a relatively short journey and we were soon installed in a nice room at the Plantation Inn, where we looked forward to two days of relaxation, and where we could unwind before starting our long trip home. The Plantation Inn was a very interesting place. In the old days, when there had been a large German presence in the South Pacific, it had been a family home. It was a very large colonial-style house, set in the most beautifully cultivated gardens. Now it had been converted into a restaurant and guesthouse by none other than Adrianne and Malu. The Waterfront hotel had been reduced to a pile of ashes in April, but now, several months later, the phoenix had risen again, albeit in a different location, in this beautiful house outside the town. It was a wonderful spot for us to spend a few days of rest and recuperation. The gardens were beautiful; the beds were soft; the baths were large and the water was clean and hot. Best of all, the food was wonderful, made all the more attractive by the total absence from the menu of fish! There were no other guests at the time we were there. It was like having a second honeymoon.

Sadly, as we were later to learn, the enterprise did not survive for long. It was just too far out of town. The intended customers would not travel so far and it was forced to close. Still, for us it had been a wonderful few days.

After a couple of days in this paradise, we were up in the morning, bright-eyed and bushy-tailed.

We headed straight into town and to the bank to change our few Samoan tala into real money, something we would be able to use outside Samoa. The manager came out to wish us farewell and then, as an afterthought, he enquired when we were flying.

We said that it would be that same afternoon. "In that case," he said, "you would be well advised to go straight to the airline office – immediately." He gave no reason, just "Go!" We left the bank with a deep sense of foreboding and almost ran to the nearby office of Polynesian Airways. There was already a crowd of people standing around, all looking at strips of paper. What could be wrong? We soon found out. It seemed that an incoming plane had come in to land with only one wheel down and had crashed on to the runway. Fortunately none of the passengers had been killed. Pushing our way inside the office and finding an airline official, we explained that we worked for the Prime Minister and that, if he checked with the P.M.'s office he would find that it was essential for us to leave Samoa as soon as possible. Better still, they should phone Terry Svensen's office. That was just around the corner and everyone knew and trusted him. We realised that we had been stretching the truth just a little, but it seemed to do the trick. A little later the official returned and advised us that we would be on the first plane out. That was the good news. The bad news was that no one knew when that would be. "In the meantime," he said, "go away! Do you need a docket?" After he had explained that this meant a docket for a hotel room, we thanked him, but said no, we thought not. We telephoned Fritz and told him what had happened. He just laughed. No one, but no one, would accept the dockets. They were worthless. "You just come here to the hotel," he said. "It's no problem."

The Inseln Fehmarn Hotel was wonderful; all mod-cons, and all of them working! There was even the offer of a car. Just as we were settling in, the telephone rang with an invitation to a party that night. It was to be a private family affair and Fritz hoped that we would be able to attend.

There would be a few other people there. Our resolution to concentrate on 'rest and relaxation' immediately went out the window and we accepted with alacrity.

The 'few other people' turned out to be an understatement. There were at least 100 guests at the party, relatives from all over the South Pacific region, with some even flown in from America. We had never seen anything like it.

The large swimming pool had been floored over, and tables and chairs set up. The variety of food was hard to describe. It was reminiscent of an MGM portrayal of a Roman orgy. At one end of the room suckling pigs were being spit-roasted and seafood of every description was laid out on the tables. At the other end were all kinds of birds, roast, broiled and baked. The sweets were too numerous to mention and the wines and spirits flowed like water. After nearly a year of living on a diet of fish and coconut milk, it was almost more than we could take in, in every sense. Sue and I were given the royal treatment. With all this conspicuous wealth, we almost felt that we were in the presence of royalty.

We were introduced to many of the guests and were surprised to find that one member of the extended family was a senior police officer, who had attended the Police Training College in our home city of Wakefield. It really was a small world!

Full of food, wine and good wishes, we retired to bed; a bed which was covered in crisp white sheets, clean and ironed – what bliss, for both of us!

The following morning we returned to the airline office hoping for news of progress. There we learned the story of how the plane had crashed into the runway. When it had landed at Tonga, two stowaways had squeezed themselves into the plane's wheel recesses. They obviously knew very little about aeroplanes and one had been caught in the mechanism as soon as the wheels had retracted. The other had died of exposure during the flight. On arrival at Samoa, the captain had been unable to lower the undercarriage, so the plane had crashed.

Upolu had only one fire engine for the entire island and there was no adequate lifting gear anywhere on Samoa. To make things worse, Samoa now had no viable credit rating with any other country. It was difficult to see how the crashed plane would ever be removed. It did not take us long to reach the conclusion that we were likely to miss our connection. We had elected to fly home via the Cook Islands, staying there for a two-week holiday. The plan was to then pick up the Air New Zealand flight for the journey back to the U.K. Now it seemed there would be no flights either into or out of Apia until the runway was cleared and another plane sorted out. In view of the country's financial situation, we could not envisage that this would be in the very near future. We decided that, in the meantime, we had better phone Steve to let him know what was going on.

We realised that we were very lucky. None of the hotels would accept a docket issued by Polynesian Airways. They knew that they would never be reimbursed. Therefore any passenger requiring a room had to pay 'up front'. We, at least, had Fritz's offer of a bed. As the Samoan proverb puts it, 'one true friend is worth any number of bankrupt airlines!'

As it turned out, just as we returned to the hotel, we received a message to visit the office of Air New Zealand. Whether it was due to the support of the Prime Minister's Office, to Terry's efforts, or just to our brazen effrontery, we shall never know, but we were immediately issued with documents allocating us seats on the first plane to fly out of Samoa. Apparently this would be an A.N.Z. flight to Auckland. What's more they offered us free hotel accommodation and breakfast while we were in New Zealand.

We stayed in the Inseln Fehmarn Hotel for a couple of days, by which time we had a good grasp of the situation. Air New Zealand knew all about the shenanigans that had been going on in the finances of Polynesian Airways and they had now repeated their offer to take over the airline, including its debts, if the entire board of directors resigned immediately. It took Polynesian Airways a couple of days to swallow this rather bitter pill, and their reluctance was shared by most of Samoa's members of parliament. After all, they had all been using it as their personal flying service, receiving free flights on demand.

While still waiting for firm news on developments, we received an invitation to visit the Manager of Air New Zealand based in Apia. It's marvellous what a little name-dropping will do! From him, we learned that arrangements had been made for a Hercules aircraft to fly in some lifting gear, so as to clear the damaged plane from the runway. The Hercules was the only plane with the lifting capacity and the necessary ability for short take off and landing. After that the next plane to arrive at Apia would be the one which would take us to Auckland, where we would stay until we boarded our flight to the Cook Islands. We would have to shorten our stay there, but a little side trip to Auckland, would more than compensate for this.

Steve arrived at the hotel in his new bus. He was taking it for a trial run. We piled in and off we went to pick up Ava's family. After driving through all the neighbouring villages we eventually arrived at Ava's house, where, surprise, surprise, Sue and I ended up cooking lunch for all of them and then preparing a dinner party for later that evening. They responded in the usual Samoan fashion, by all falling asleep on their eating mats. Sue developed a migraine!

By the Thursday afternoon everything was sorted out. Our flight tickets had been re-validated; the runway had been cleared; and we were due to fly out at 2.00 a.m. on the following morning, Friday 16th September 1994. By the time we arrived in Auckland it would be Saturday morning and we would stay there for just over a day, flying out on the Sunday afternoon. After a relatively short flight, we would arrive at Raratonga on Saturday 17th September! It was all rather confusing. Thanks to the International Date Line, we would have two Saturdays and two Sundays that week. Certainly my digital wristwatch never knew what day it was the entire time we were in the South Pacific!

Our short stop-over in New Zealand allowed us to get to know Auckland quite well. I think we must have walked the city from top to bottom.

Our first impression of Raratonga in the Cook Islands was that it was expensive. Terry and Luanna had warned us that it would not be cheap, but the prices were horrendous. We now realised that the enforced curtailment of our stay by the events in Apia was really a blessing. Of course it was wonderful to have electricity and hot water 'on tap' and we appreciated beds with crisp and freshly laundered sheets each day, but it put a great strain on our limited budget.

The food was beautiful; we tried a lasagne, which was so light it was unbelievable. The tomato covering was made with real tomatoes and fresh cream; even the garlic bread had a lightness as if it had been made with a cake mix.

Whilst we had been staying in the Plantation Inn, Miss Adrianne had given us a note of introduction to a friend of hers, also a New Zealander, who lived on Raratonga and was a dealer in black pearls. That's where we headed on the day after our arrival. What an interesting guy! He obviously loved black pearls and his enthusiasm was infectious. He explained to us, in great detail, how they were produced and how to assess their quality. Then, after a couple of hours, he sent us off into town to look at the jewellery shops, to see how the pearls were mounted. The gold work was just breathtaking. I had never seen anything so delicate at home. Sue had her sketch pad and was busy making notes and drawings of her favourite pieces.

The following day we returned to the New Zealander and selected two beautiful black pearls.

While Sue had been busy choosing her pearls, I had been in conversation with the dealer and, as a result, obtained from him an introduction to one of the consultants at the local hospital. That's how, on the following morning, we came to be walking in the sunshine, up to the hospital. It was a real eye-opener. It was as if we were in a first-rate European hospital. We found the rest of the island equally impressive. It was so clean and the people looked well-dressed and happy; so unlike the Samoans. Even the children were clean and neatly dressed. It must have all been to do with the relative affluence of the Cook Islanders, as they and the Samoans all have the same Polynesian origins.

We walked a lot, and when we were exhausted with that, we sunbathed and rested. Our apartment was set in a small complex with lovely gardens and areas of relaxation. It was idyllic. Sue responded to the place and to the atmosphere. She was looking younger by the day, laughing and blushing. It was wonderful to see. It was all so different from Samoa. It was a place to which we would both love to return and, with hindsight, it was probably no more expensive than Samoa, but with so much more to offer.

We submerged ourselves in the luxury of it all. For supper we had crab (and we didn't have to get the permission of the Elders!) – and what crab. Even the claws had teeth. With toasted cheese and spaghetti it was delicious.

On our final evening we strolled down to the waterside, to a small place called Trader Jacks, where we had fish and chips, with salt and vinegar and pickled onions, all served in a newspaper. We finally felt that we were really on our way home.

So now it is time to close what is my story, <u>Max's Story</u>, as I saw it and recall it. It had been a year to remember, a year that I shall never forget.

———————— ,, ————————

P.S. We brought back from Samoa a rather large wooden carving; someone whom we knew had carved it for Steve's bus. We had loved it so much that we purchased it to bring home to put on our wall. It accompanied us safely all the way to London; there it was stolen from out of our heap of luggage as we waited for the bus to bring us from London to Wakefield. No one could steal our memories!